Lactose-Free Cooking

Recipes for

People Sensitive to

Dairy Products

by

Arlene Burlant, RD

ISBN: 0-9626941-0-X

Library of Congress Catalog Card Number: 90-93143

Published By Lockley Publishers, Inc., Wayne, New Jersey

Printed in the United States of America by BookCrafters, Inc., Chelsea, Michigan

Book Design and Typesetting by Office Extensions, Mountain Lakes, New Jersey

Current Printing (last digit)
9 8 7 6 5 4 3 2 1

No comment or recipe in this book is to be construed as a substitute for advice from a physician or registered dietitian: medical and dietary questions pertaining to lactose intolerance, dietary issues or, in general, any aspect of personal health should be discussed with a physician and/or registered dietitian.

Mention of brand names is for illustration only, not to be taken as a recommendation; nor is any list of manufacturers for a product to be taken as complete, since such a list is for illustration only.

This Book is Dedicated to

Anita and Morris,

Without Whose Dietary Problems

It Would Not Have Been Written

CONTENTS

INTRODUCTION

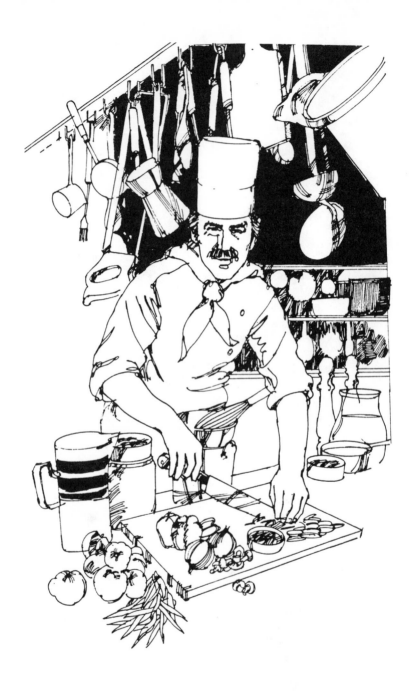

Lactose Intolerance

One of the most important nutrients in milk is the natural sugar lactose. To digest lactose, the body normally produces an enzyme called lactase, the function of which is to break down lactose to simpler sugars. When the body does not manufacture this enzyme in sufficient quantity, digestion of milk and milk products occurs with difficulty: a lactase-deficient -- or lactose intolerant -- person may have symptoms such as gas, cramps, and/or diarrhea when he or she ingests dairy products because the unmodified sugar remains in the small intestine for too long a time.

Certain foods, including peas, lima beans, beets, liver, sweetbreads and brains, contain glycosides which are degraded to lactose; persons sensitive to lactose may need to avoid these foods.

About three-quarters of the adults in the world exhibit lactose intolerance; in the United States alone there are at least 30 million such individuals. Lactose intolerance is uncommon in young children.

Some lactose intolerance may occur in persons with a history of intestinal problems such as intestinal infection; as a result of gastric surgery; as a result of other enzyme deficiencies; with use of medications such as antibiotics or some anti-inflammatory drugs; and in some instances with exposure to therapeutic doses of high energy radiation.

A less common problem with dairy products is the allergic reaction to the protein in cow's milk. A small fraction of infants exhibit this sensitivity. For the infants allergic to cow's milk, there are formulas based on protein from soybeans; for infants allergic to both soybean and cow's milk protein, there are special preparations made from predigested milk protein. Fortunately, such immune-derived allergies usually disappear before the age of three.

It is important generally to consult a physician and/or a registered dietitian for advice or information about health and dietary matters, but it is especially important in matters related to lactose intolerance since, in a small number of instances, there may be an underlying intestinal disease accompanying the lactose problem.

Milk and Milk Products

Most lactose-intolerant individuals adjust their diets by restricting use of milk products, i.e., limiting intake of milk, cheese and ice cream. But elimination of lactose-containing foods such as milk and cheeses may generate other problems, since such foods are important sources of nutrients such as calcium, vitamins A, D and the B group.

Some suggestions to consider before reducing intake of these critical foods: Milk in smaller portions (4 ounces) more often throughout the day and milk taken with solid foods may reduce or eliminate discomfort due to lactose. Whole milk may be tolerated better than lowfat milk; tolerance for cocoa and chocolate milk may be better than that for unflavored milk. And most aged cheeses, like Swiss and Cheddar, because of their low lactose content, may be accepted.

Lactose-reduced milk and milk to which lactases, such as Lactaid, are added at mealtime may improve tolerance to milk; tolerance to cultured buttermilk and sweet acidophilus milk is similar to that for whole milk. Lactose-reduced milks can be used in place of unmodified milk in virtually all recipes.

Yogurts often are tolerated because yogurt cultures produce the needed enzyme lactase; yogurts which are not pasteurized (since pasteurization inactivates the enzyme) often may be used by milk-sensitive individuals. Non-pasteurized yogurts include Dannon, Columbo, Yoplait, Kraft and Breyers. A cheese substitute can be created by filtering the solids from most such yogurts using a fine strainer available for this purpose in kitchenware shops.

Lactose-reduced cottage cheese is available from Friendship and Lactaid; low-lactose American cheese is offered by Lactaid. A number of companies, in addition to the examples given, offer lactose-reduced cheeses.

Lactose-Free Foods

The incorporation of substitute dairy products into the diet often is a good way to deal with lactose sensitivity. A few examples of some popular substitute dairy items are given below:

- **Tofu** -- a non-dairy product made from soybeans -- is a protein-complete, digestible food. An 8 ounce serving provides a substantial fraction of an adult's daily protein and calcium requirements. There is on the market a non-dairy "yogurt" called Jofu, which is tofu-based and fruit flavored.

- **Lactose-free** "ice creams" are manufactured by Loft (Tofulite); TofuTime (Tofutti); and Farm Foods (Ice Bean sandwiches).

- **Soymilks** -- also derived from soybeans -- are nutritionally quite complete, supplying many of the important nutrients present in milk without the latter's lactose. Many non-dairy creams, ice creams and shortening (margarines) are made from lactose-free soy (or other vegetable oils) suitably flavored. Soymilks are available from many sources, including Eden Foods, Worthington Foods, and Loma Linda Foods.

- **Milk, cream and whipping cream substitutes,** based on vegetable oil: these include Hunt's Reddi-Whip; Rich's Rich Whip; Rich's Coffee Rich and Poly Rich; Whitehouse's Presto Whip; Cool Whip; Carnation's Coffee-mate; and Formagg's "sour cream".

- **Milk-free margarines,** made from vegetable oils, are offered by Diet Imperial, Mazola, Manischewitz, Mar-Parv, Mother's, Fleischmann's and Weight Watchers.

- **Non-dairy cheeses,** made from vegetable oils, are available from Formagg (mozzarella, provolone, ricotta, cream, cheddar and parmesan); Che Soya (cheddar, Swiss); Mrs. Margareten (mozzarella, parmesan, Swiss, cream, Monterey Jack); Soya-Kass (tofu-based cream cheese); and Parvcheezy (cheddar).

Often, substitute dairy products are not simple replacements for the milk-containing item: for example, many of the cream substitutes cannot be sufficiently whipped; milk-free margarines may brown when heated excessively; yogurt cheeses are heat sensitive; non-dairy cheeses do not always taste just like their natural counterparts, exhibit quite different textures and usually are best used at the end of the recipe after the other ingredients have been cooked; soy-based milks sometimes add color to the final dish and may not be heated to too high temperatures; when substituting soymilk for cream, it may be advisable to replace 1 tablespoon of the soy products with 1 tablespoon vegetable oil; soymilks are formulated with different kinds and concentrations of ingredients (e.g., flavorings and sweeteners) and may respond differently in recipes; tofu, when overcooked, becomes rubbery; and enzyme-treated milks (those with Lactaid, for example) are sweeter than unmodified milk, so less sweetener is needed when used in recipes. It is important to test any new recipe you may develop to ensure it meets your taste and texture requirements.

Note that while non-dairy cream and whipped cream is used in some recipes for variety and flavor, these may contain significant amounts of sugar and may contain saturated fats.

It is wise to read carefully the labels of these substitute dairy products and to choose ones that are enriched with important nutrients and those with the least amount of saturated oils such as coconut, palm and palm kernel -- the so-called tropical oils.

Substitute dairy products for consumers are being introduced at a rapid rate; check the food store for the newer varieties.

A Balanced Diet

When maintaining a lactose-reduced or lactose-free diet, it is critical to ensure an adequate supply of the nutrients lost as a consequence of the reduced intake of milk and milk products.

Calcium is one of the most important elements for proper growth and functioning of the human body. The following Table presents the daily allowances, as recommended by the National Research Council:

TABLE I.   DAILY CALCIUM REQUIREMENTS

	Age	mg Calcium
Infants	to 6 months	360
	6 months to 1 year	540
Children	1 – 10 years	800
Adolescents	11 – 18 years	1,200
Adults	19 years and over	800
Pregnant or breast-feeding women	under 19 years	1,600
	over 19 years	1,200

But milk furnishes other nutrients as well:

TABLE II.   PERCENT OF DAILY NUTRIENT REQUIREMENTS IN A CUP OF MILK

Calcium	76	Protein	34	Vitamin A	26
Vitamin D	50	Riboflavin	60	Vitamin B_{12}	60

While the nutrients in the above table occur in enzyme-treated low lactose milk products, for truly non-dairy diets, other sources are needed for an adequate supply of these dietary essentials.

- Calcium is found in leafy green vegetables such as kale, collards, canned salmon and sardines, almonds and citrus fruits.

- High protein foods include poultry, meat, fish and soy products, along with the combination (i.e., when eaten together) of pasta or bread with beans.

- Vitamin A is found in liver, dark green leafy vegetables, carrots, sweet potatoes and apricots.

- Vitamin D is in liver, eggs and fish.

- Riboflavin is found in liver, dark green leafy vegetables and whole grain foods.

- Vitamin B_{12} is in liver, fish and eggs.

Table III highlights the nutrient content of some common non-dairy foods important in lactose-free or lactose-reduced diets.

TABLE III. PERCENTAGE OF DAILY REQUIREMENTS OF NUTRIENTS IN NON-DAIRY FOODS

	Calcium	Protein	Vit A	Vit D	Riboflavin	Vit B12
Sardines, 3 ounces[1]	411	43	5	64	15	250
Salmon, can 3 ounces[1]	25	36	4	106	13	197
Spinach, ½ cup, cooked[2]	17	8	185	0	12	0
Meat, chuck/ground, 3 ounces	1	44	1	0	13	80
Liver, 3 ounces	1	43	940	9	270	2000
Fish, perch, 3 ounces	15	42	1	0	8	40
Carrots, ½ cup	3	2	479	0	3	0
Whole grain, pumpernickel, 2 slices	6	12	0	0	26	0
Almonds, 1 ounces	10	9	0	0	15	0
Eggs, 1 large	4	13	7	7	12	20
Egg substitute, 1½ ounces	3	12	25	2	11	1
Soymilk[3] (a soybean product) 6 ounces	10	15	0	0	8	0
Tofu[3] (soybean curd), 4 ounces	8	12	0	0	6	0

[1] With bones. [2] Not all the calcium in spinach may be available for metabolism; other green vegetables high in calcium and Vitamin A are collards, kale, beet greens, turnip greens and broccoli. [3] These values are for a particular soy product from one manufacturer; other sources may yield different values.

Recipes

The recipes collected in this book reflect the information described in the preceding pages and are based on lactose-free products or those foods generally tolerated by lactose-sensitive individuals.

Some ethnic groups use little or no milk in cooking so these are good sources of lactose-free meals as well as ideas for new dishes: Chinese and Japanese meat dishes are virtually milk-free; Jewish kosher-labelled meat-containing and pareve foods contain no dairy products; Indian recipes use almost no milk (but watch for those calling for milk curd); and many Spanish dishes are milk-free. Of course, lactose-reduced milk may be substituted for unmodified milk in most dishes.

Thus a number of recipes, normally using dairy products have been reformulated to incorporate dairy substitutes and fruit juice for milk, where applicable; many recipes have been redesigned to eliminate both dairy products and their substitutes; and for convenience and completeness, where a desirable nutrient is present, some popular normally lactose-free recipes are included.

The recipes conform, as much as possible, to the dietary guidelines set forth by the Surgeon General's Report on Nutrition and Health aimed at reducing, in some measure, the risks of heart attacks, strokes and cancer. These guidelines include reduction of saturated and total fat (for example, by using pureed vegetables to thicken soups, thus replacing heavy cream); use of fish in place of meat; use of more high fiber foods; reduction of egg yolk and egg yolk products (by using egg whites or egg substitutes and egg-free mayonnaise); less organ meats; and inclusion of complex carbohydrates (breads, pasta, fruits and vegetables) in daily diets.

- The recipes in this book, to a large extent, use dairy-free egg whites or yolk-free egg products in place of whole eggs (Egg Beaters is one example of such a product).

- Low-fat ingredients (cheeses, mayonnaise, yogurt and meats) are used when available.

- All purpose flour is used throughout the book.

- Non-stick skillets and/or non-stick sprays are used when sauteing.

- It is assumed that 1 loaf of bread yields 16 slices.

- When thickening foods, 1 tablespoon cornstarch plus 1 tablespoon cold water thickens 1 cup liquid; 3 tablespoons flour plus 2 tablespoons vegetable oil thickens 2 cups liquid.

- When beating egg whites, use utensils free from grease, and at room temperature; egg whites should be completely free from yolk particles. The first stage in the beating process produces soft peaks which are fluffy and creamy; the second stage produces peaks which hold their shape but still are moist (for mousses, souffles and puddings); the third stage produces stiff and dry peaks (used for pie toppings).

- Common substitutes for milk in virtually all recipes include water, fruit juice, soymilk, non-dairy cream diluted with water and lactose-reduced whole milk.

- Salt has been omitted from many recipes, with the understanding that it may be added as desired; low-salt meat and chicken bouillon are used where possible.

- Abbreviations used in this book include:

  gm = grams   mg = milligrams

- Some convenient equivalent measures include:

  3 teaspoons = 1 tablespoon
  4 tablespoons = ¼ cup
  16 tablespoons = 1 cup
  1 cup = ½ pint (8 ounces)

- Temperatures are given in °Fahrenheit

- Most meat exchanges in this book are based on medium-fat meat, for which 7 gm protein and 5 gm fat are taken as one meat exchange.

- Serving suggestions (the statement, "serve with rice or noodles", for example) are not incorporated in the NUTRIENTS and EXCHANGES values.

DIPS

Many dips contain cream, sour cream or cheese; the ones described in this section are based on vegetable and soy products. They can be served with vegetables, crackers, pita bread or toast points.

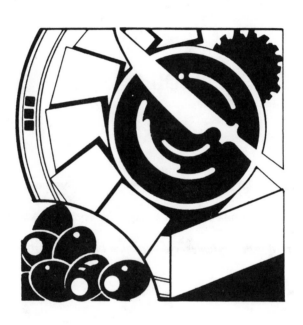

EGGPLANT DIP

3 cups

1 large eggplant
¼ cup olive oil
1 teaspoon minced garlic
1½ cups peeled diced tomatoes, drained
2 tablespoons lemon juice
2 tablespoons tomato paste
¼ cup finely chopped onion
pepper to taste

Peel eggplant and cut into ½ inch cubes. Heat olive oil in a skillet and saute the eggplant with the garlic; stir occasionally until eggplant is soft enough to mash with spoon. Remove eggplant and cool. Add diced tomatoes to mashed eggplant together with remaining ingredients; stir.

NUTRIENTS, per tablespoon:

Calories 13	Protein 0.1 gm	Carbohydrates 2 gm
Calcium 1 mg	Total fat 1 gm	Saturated fat 0.2 gm

EXCHANGES, per tablespoon: free

GUACAMOLE DIP

2 cups

2 tablespoons minced onions
1 large tomato, peeled and finely chopped
1 teaspoon minced green chilies
2 tablespoons lemon juice
¼ teaspoon chopped garlic
2 large, ripe mashed avocados

Combine all ingredients except avocado and let stand about an hour in refrigerator; mash avocado before serving and combine with other ingredients.

NUTRIENTS, per tablespoon:

Calories 22	Protein 0.3	Carbohydrates 2 gm
Calcium 2 mg	Total fat 2 gm	Saturated fat 0.3 gm

EXCHANGES, per tablespoon: ½ fat

HOUMMOUS DIP   1½ cups

12 ounces of tehina (a blend of chick peas and sesame paste)
1 teaspoon lemon juice
¼ teaspoon paprika

Blend the first two ingredients; garnish with paprika.

NUTRIENTS, per tablespoon:

Calories 38	Protein 1.7 gm	Carbohydrates 2.6 gm
Calcium 80 mg	Total fat 3 gm	Saturated fat 0.3 gm

EXCHANGES, per tablespoon: ½ fat

ONION DIP   3 cups

½ cup olive oil
½ cup water
3 tablespoons lemon juice
1 tablespoon wine vinegar
1¾ pounds tofu
1 envelope of dehydrated onion soup mix

Combine the liquid ingredients in a blender. Add the tofu, piece by piece, until it is all blended, and the mixture smooth. Turn into a bowl, and stir in the onion soup mix. Refrigerate for 1 hour before serving.

<u>NUTRIENTS</u>, per tablespoon:

Calories 27	Protein 1 gm	Carbohydrates 0.3 gm
Calcium 10 mg	Total fat 3 gm	Saturated fat 0.2 gm

<u>EXCHANGES</u>, per tablespoon: ½ fat

BEAN DIP   *2 cups*

1½ cups cooked black or red beans
3 tablespoons lemon juice
2 tablespoons olive oil
½ teaspoon crushed garlic
8 ounces tofu

In a food processor or blender, blend all ingredients until creamy, adding the tofu gradually to the other ingredients. Serve garnished with parsley.

<u>NUTRIENTS</u>, per tablespoon:

Calories 15	Protein 1 gm	Carbohydrates 1 gm
Calcium 6 mg	Total fat 1 gm	Saturated fat 0.1 gm

<u>EXCHANGES</u>, per tablespoon: free

CURRY DIP   *2 cups*

¼ cup olive oil
2 tablespoons lemon juice
½ teaspoon Worcestershire sauce
½ teaspoon curry powder
½ teaspoon dry mustard
¼ teaspoon crushed garlic
12 ounces tofu

Combine all ingredients, except tofu, in a blender. With the blender on, add the tofu in small pieces until blended and the mixture smooth.

NUTRIENTS, per tablespoon:

Calories 22	Protein 1 gm	Carbohydrates 0.3 gm
Calcium 13 mg	Total fat 2 gm	Saturated fat 0.3 gm

EXCHANGES, per tablespoon: ½ fat

SMOKED SALMON DIP   *1 cup*

5 ounces smoked salmon, shredded
1/3 cup non-dairy cream
pepper to taste

Blend all ingredients in a blender until smooth.

NUTRIENTS, per tablespoon:

Calories 42	Protein 5 gm	Carbohydrates 1 gm
Calcium 21 mg	Total fat 2 gm	Saturated fat 0.3 gm

EXCHANGES, not applicable

MOCK CREAM CHEESE   *1 cup*

1 cup low-lactose cottage cheese, drained
2 tablespoons vegetable oil

Blend the ingredients in a blender until creamy. The flavor can be
modified by adding 1 tablespoon of finely chopped green pepper and
1 tablespoon of chopped onion.

NUTRIENTS, per tablespoon:

Calories 26	Protein 2 gm	Carbohydrates 1 gm
Calcium 9 mg	Total fat 2 gm	Saturated fat 0.4 gm

EXCHANGES, per tablespoon: ½ fat

BREADS & MUFFINS

Bread is a source of carbohydrates and B vitamins. For persons on dairy-free diets the protein in milk products is not available; it is important, therefore to recall that beans and peas supply amino acids that complement those in grains, making this combination of foods an additional source of the needed protein.

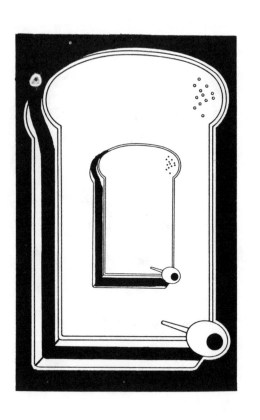

FAT-FREE WHITE BREAD   *1 loaf*

1 package active dry yeast
¼ cup warm water
1 teaspoon sugar
¼ teaspoon salt
1 cup orange juice
2½ cups white flour
¼ teaspoon baking soda
2 tablespoons cornmeal

Mix yeast with warm water and sugar; let stand for 5 minutes. When yeast is softened, add salt and juice. Stir in 1 cup of flour to which the baking soda has been added. Beat well for 2 minutes. Stir in rest of flour to make a stiff batter. Spoon into 5 x 9 inch loaf pan that has been sprayed with cooking spray and sprinkled with cornmeal. Sprinkle top with cornmeal. Cover, let rise in warm place for 45 minutes or until doubled. Bake in a preheated 400 degree oven for 25 minutes.

NUTRIENTS, per slice:

Calories 63	Protein 2 gm	Carbohydrates 14 gm
Calcium 3 mg	Total fat 0.2 gm	Saturated fat 0.03 gm

EXCHANGES, per slice: 1 bread

WHITE BREAD I   *2 loaves*

6 cups all purpose flour
2 packages active dry yeast
2 tablespoons sugar
¼ teaspoon salt
3 tablespoons non-dairy softened margarine
2 cups hot water
1 teaspoon cooking oil

Combine 1 cup flour, undissolved yeast, sugar and salt in a large bowl; stir well, then add margarine and hot water. Beat with an electric mixer for 2 minutes. Add another cup of flour and beat on high speed for 1 minute until dough is thick and elastic. Add remaining flour, stirring it in with a wooden spoon; place on a floured board. Knead for 10 minutes or until dough is smooth. Let rise 20 minutes.

Punch down and shape dough into two loaves; place each loaf in a 5 x 9 inch greased loaf pan; brush top lightly with cooking oil. Cover pan loosely with a towel; allow dough to rise for about 1 hour. Bake bread in a preheated 400° oven for 30 to 40 minutes.

NUTRIENTS, per slice:

Calories 90	Protein 2 gm	Carbohydrates 17 gm
Calcium 4 mg	Total fat 1 gm	Saturated fat 0.2 gm

EXCHANGES, per slice: 1 bread

WHITE BREAD II   *2 loaves*

7 cups flour
2 packages dry yeast
3 tablespoons sugar
½ tablespoon salt
½ cup instant mashed potatoes
2 cups very hot tap water
¼ cup non-dairy margarine

Combine thoroughly in mixer bowl 2 cups flour, dry yeast, sugar and salt. Mix instant potatoes with hot water and margarine; add to dry ingredients; beat for 2 minutes at medium speed. Add 2 cups flour; beat on high speed for another 2 minutes; stir in remaining flour with a spoon. Turn out on a floured board; knead until smooth and elastic (8 to 10 minutes). Place in greased bowl, cover with towel and let rise in warm place until doubled in bulk (1 hour); punch dough down. Turn out on floured board, cover and let rise 15 minutes.

Grease two 5 x 9 inch loaf pans. Divide dough in half and shape into 2 loaves; place in pans, cover, and let rise until double in bulk (1 hour). Bake in preheated 400° oven for 25 to 30 minutes.

NUTRIENTS, per slice:

Calories 107	Protein 2.6 gm	Carbohydrates 20 gm
Calcium 5 mg	Total fat 2 gm	Saturated fat 0.3 gm

EXCHANGES, per slice: 1 bread; ½ fat

RYE BREAD   *2 loaves*

6 cups rye flour
2 packages dry yeast
½ cup instant mashed potatoes
½ teaspoon salt
2 cups hot tap water
½ cup sugar
¼ cup salad oil

In large mixer bowl thoroughly mix 2 cups flour with yeast. Add instant mashed potatoes to hot water; whip lightly with fork and add salt. Combine oil with potatoes and water mixture; add to dry ingredients. Beat 2 minutes at medium speed of mixer, scraping bowl occasionally. Add 2 cups flour. Beat at high speed 2 minutes, scraping bowl occasionally. Stir in remaining 2 cups flour (or enough to make a stiff dough). Sprinkle bread board with rye flour. Turn dough out and knead until smooth and elastic (8 to 10 minutes). Place dough in greased bowl; cover with a towel and let rise in warm place until double in bulk (about 1½ hours).

Punch down dough and shape into 2 loaves. Cover and let rise until double in bulk (30 to 45 minutes). Divide dough into 2 halves, place each in a greased 5 x 9 inch loaf pan and bake in a preheated 350° oven for 40 minutes.

NUTRIENTS, per slice:

Calories 93	Protein 2.5 gm	Carbohydrates 17 gm
Calcium 7.8 mg	Total fat 2.1 gm	Saturated fat 0.3 gm

EXCHANGES, not applicable

CORN BREAD   *9 servings*

1½ cups corn meal
3 tablespoons rice flour
¼ teaspoon salt
1 tablespoon sugar
1 teaspoon baking powder
1½ cups water
3 eggs
2 tablespoons salad oil

Grease 8 inch square baking pan. Sift together dry ingredients. Add water, eggs, and oil; mix just until dry ingredients are moistened. Pour into pan; bake in a preheated 450° oven for 20 minutes.

NUTRIENTS, per serving:

Calories 130	Protein 2 gm	Carbohydrates 16 gm
Calcium 11 mg	Total fat 5 gm	Saturated fat 1 gm

EXCHANGES, per serving: 1 bread; 1 fat

OATMEAL BREAD

2 loaves

2 cups oatmeal
2½ cups hot water
½ cup molasses
¼ tablespoon salt
¼ cup salad oil
6 cups flour
2 packages dry yeast

Pour hot water over oatmeal. Add molasses, salt and salad oil; mix. In mixer bowl combine thoroughly 2 cups flour and dry yeast. Add oatmeal mixture; beat 2 minutes at medium speed scraping bowl. Add 1 cup flour and beat another 2 minutes at high speed, scraping bowl frequently. Stir in remaining flour with spoon. Knead on lightly floured board 8 to 10 minutes until dough is smooth and elastic. Return dough to greased bowl. Cover with towel and let rise until double in bulk (1 hour).

Grease two 5 x 9 inch loaf pans. Punch down dough. Shape into 2 loaves and place in pans. Cover and let rise until double in bulk (1 hour). Bake 45 minutes in a preheated 375° oven.

NUTRIENTS, per slice:

Calories 135	Protein 3.2 gm	Carbohydrates 25 gm
Calcium 15 mg	Total fat 2 gm	Saturated fat 0.2 gm

EXCHANGES, not applicable

MULTI-GRAIN BREAD   *1 loaf*

1 package active dry yeast
½ cup lukewarm water
2 tablespoons molasses
2 tablespoons honey
1 tablespoon oil
1 cup orange juice
¾ cup whole wheat flour
¾ cup rye flour
¼ cup rolled oats (not instant)
¼ cup cornmeal
½ teaspoon salt
2 cups white flour

Mix yeast, water, molasses, honey and oil. Add orange juice and stir well, making sure yeast is complete dissolved. Add whole wheat flour, rye flour, oats, cornmeal, salt and 1 cup of white flour. Stir until thoroughly mixed. Cover with towel; let rise in warm place until doubled (about 1½ hours).

Sprinkle board with 1 cup white flour and knead into dough, adding more flour if dough is still sticky. When all flour has been absorbed, knead until smooth. Shape into loaf; put in 5 x 9 inch loaf pan; cover and let rise in warm place until doubled in bulk (about 45 minutes). Bake bread in a 400° preheated oven for 20 minutes, then lower temperature to 350° and bake for 30 minutes longer.

NUTRIENTS, per slice:

Calories 146	Protein 4 gm	Carbohydrates 31 gm
Calcium 13 mg	Total fat 1.3 gm	Saturated fat 0.2 gm

EXCHANGES, not applicable

BOSTON BROWN BREAD

1 loaf

¾ *cup rye flour*
¾ *cup cornmeal*
¾ *cup whole wheat flour*
2 *teaspoons baking soda*
½ *teaspoon salt*
1½ *cups mashed tofu*
1 *tablespoon water*
1 *cup soy milk*
½ *cup molasses*
1 *tablespoon lemon juice*

Mix together the dry ingredients in a large bowl. In a blender, puree the tofu with the water. Mix together the tofu puree with the remaining liquid ingredients. Stir the liquid ingredients into the dry ingredients and mix well. Oil a 5 x 9 inch loaf pan and fill with batter no more than two-thirds full. Seal the top tightly with foil. Place the covered pan on a steamer rack in a large pot that is at least 3 inches taller than the mold. Pour boiling water into the pot until it reaches a height halfway up the pan; cover and steam for 1 to 1½ hours, keeping the water boiling; add more, if necessary, to maintain a constant height of water around the pan. Remove the pan from the pot and take off the foil cover. Set the pan in a 300° pre-heated over for 10 minutes to dry the bread slightly. Serve at room temperature.

NUTRIENTS, per slice:

Calories 70	Protein 1 mg	Carbohydrates 15 gm
Calcium 17 mg	Total fat 1 gm	Saturated fat 0.1 gm

EXCHANGES, not applicable

ORANGE NUT BREAD   *1 loaf*

2¼ cups oat flour
4 teaspoons baking powder
¼ teaspoon baking soda
¾ cup sugar
¼ teaspoon salt
1 cup chopped walnuts
2 tablespoons salad oil
¾ cup orange juice
1 tablespoon grated orange rind

Sift together dry ingredients. Add nuts, oil, orange juice and orange
rind; stir until dry ingredients are moistened; pour into lightly greased
5 x 9 loaf pan. Bake in a 350° preheated oven for 1 hour.

NUTRIENTS, per slice:

Calories 144	Protein 4 gm	Carbohydrates 16 gm
Calcium 12 mg	Total fat 2 gm	Saturated fat 0.5 gm

EXCHANGES, not applicable

PUMPKIN BREAD   *2 loaves*

½ cup salad oil
1 cup sugar
1 cup firmly packed brown sugar
2 cups (1 lb) canned pumpkin
2½ cups flour
2 teaspoons baking soda
2 teaspoons pumpkin pie spice
¼ teaspoon salt
½ cup chopped dates

Grease two 5 x 9 inch loaf pans. Combine oil, sugars and pumpkin in mixing bowl. Beat well. Add sifted dry ingredients. Mix just until all dry ingredients are moistened, fold in dates. Pour batter into pans and bake in a 350° preheated over for 1 hour.

NUTRIENTS, per slice:

Calories 120	Protein 1 gm	Carbohydrates 22 gm
Calcium 13 mg	Total fat 4 gm	Saturated fat 0.3 gm

EXCHANGES, not applicable

ROLLS   *2 dozen*

3 ¼ cups flour
1 package dry yeast
½ cup sugar
½ teaspoon salt
2 tablespoons instant mashed potatoes
½ cup non-dairy margarine, melted
1 cup hot water

In mixer bowl combine thoroughly 1 cup flour, dry yeast, sugar and salt. Add potatoes and margarine to dry ingredients; add water and beat 2 minutes at medium speed, scraping side of bowl often. Add 1 cup flour and beat at high speed 2 additional minutes. Add remaining flour and mix thoroughly; cover bowl with towel and refrigerate at least 2 hours. Shape dough into rolls. Place on greased cookie sheet 2 inches apart. Let rise until double in bulk (45 minute). Bake in preheated 350° oven for 15 minutes (until lightly browned).

For sweet rolls: Divide dough in half; roll out each half to 9" x 18" rectangle. Brush with melted non-dairy margarine. Sprinkle with sugar, cinnamon and raisins. Roll up like a jelly roll; cut into 1" slices. After baking, sprinkle with powdered sugar.

NUTRIENTS, per basic roll:

Calories 90	Protein 2 gm	Carbohydrates 14 gm
Calcium 4 mg	Total fat 4 gm	Saturated fat 0.5 gm

EXCHANGES, per roll: not applicable

EXCHANGES, per sweet roll: not applicable

BAGELS   *1 dozen*

2 packages dry yeast
1½ cups warm water
3 tablespoons granulated sugar
1 teaspoon salt
1 tablespoon non-dairy margarine
4 cups all-purpose flour
2½ quarts water

Dissolve yeast in ½ cup warm water; add the rest of the water, 2 tablespoons sugar, ½ teaspoons salt, margarine and 2 cups of the flour. Beat until smooth, then add the remaining flour to make a somewhat stiff dough. Knead on a floured surface for about 10 minutes; cover with towel and let rest for 20 minutes. Roll dough to ¾ inch thickness. Cut sections with a 3-inch doughnut cutter. Place on ungreased cookie sheet, cover and let rise 20 minutes.

In a large pot, bring to a boil the remaining water, salt and sugar; drop 2-4 bagels into the water, simmer for 2 minutes on each side, drain and place on greased cookie sheet. Bake in preheated 425° oven for 20-25 minutes or until golden brown.

NUTRIENTS, per bagel:

Calories 150	Protein 4 gm	Carbohydrates 30 gm
Calcium 7 mg	Total fat 1.3 gm	Saturated fat 0.3 gm

EXCHANGES, not applicable

CHALLAH

2 loaves

6 cups flour
2 packages active dry yeast
2 cups water
2 tablespoons sugar
½ teaspoon salt
3 eggs
4 tablespoons vegetable oil

Sift the flour into a large bowl. Crumble the yeast into a small bowl; add warm water and sugar. When it bubbles (after a few minutes) add salt. Beat eggs and save 1 tablespoon to use as a glaze for the loaves; add 3 tablespoons oil and the sugar to the remaining beaten eggs and stir well. Stir egg mixture into the yeast mixture and quickly stir the combined mixture into the flour until a soft ball is formed. Knead until smooth and elastic. Place in a large bowl, brush additional oil over surface of dough, cover with towel and let rise in a warm place until double in bulk. Punch dough down and knead again. Divide the dough in half and divide each half into three parts. Form long fat ropes of the dough and braid three ropes loosely together. Repeat with second group of three ropes. Place each braid into a greased 5 x 9 inch loaf pan; let rise for ½ hour. Brush with reserved beaten egg; bake in 400° preheated oven for 45 minutes.

NUTRIENTS, per slice:

Calories 99	Protein 2.8 gm	Carbohydrates 17 gm
Calcium 6.5 mg	Total fat 2.4 gm	Saturated fat 0.4 gm

EXCHANGES, per slice: 1 bread; ½ fat

OAT BISCUITS   *1 dozen*

1 cup oat flour
3 teaspoons baking powder
¼ teaspoon salt
1 tablespoon sugar
1 tablespoon non-dairy margarine
1/3 cup cold water

Sift together dry ingredients; cut margarine into ¼ inch pieces and add to dry ingredients. All cold water; stir gently to form soft dough. Knead lightly on board dusted with oat flour. Roll to ½ inch thickness; cut with 1½ inch round cutter and place on ungreased cookie sheet. Bake in a preheated 450° oven for 15 to 20 minutes.

NUTRIENTS, per biscuit:

Calories 50	Protein 1 gm	Carbohydrates 7 gm
Calcium 66 mg	Total fat 2 gm	Saturated fat 0.3 gm

EXCHANGES, per biscuit: ½ bread; ½ fat

DATE NUT MUFFINS   *1 dozen*

1 teaspoon baking soda
1 cup chopped, pitted dates
¾ cup boiling water
¼ cup non-dairy margarine
1½ cups flour
½ cup sugar
¼ cup chopped almonds

Sprinkle baking soda over dates in mixing bowl. Add boiling water and the remaining ingredients; mix until moistened. Fill greased muffin tins two-thirds full. Bake in preheated 375° oven for 20 to 25 minutes.

NUTRIENTS, per muffin:

Calories 168	Protein 3 gm	Carbohydrates 19 gm
Calcium 34 mg	Total fat 3 gm	Saturated fat 0.3 gm

EXCHANGES, not applicable

OAT MUFFINS   *1 dozen*

2 cups oat flour
1½ teaspoons baking powder
¼ teaspoon salt
½ cup sugar
1¼ cups hot water
½ cup raisins
¼ cup vegetable oil

Sift together dry ingredients. Pour hot water over raisins; add vegetable oil, add this mixture to dry ingredients and mix until moistened. Fill greased muffin tins two-thirds full. Bake in preheated 400° oven for 25 minutes.

NUTRIENTS, per muffin:

Calories 114	Protein 2 gm	Carbohydrates 19 gm
Calcium 9 mg	Total fat 4 gm	Saturated fat 0.4 gm

EXCHANGES, not applicable

BLUEBERRY MUFFINS   *1 dozen*

2 cups all purpose flour
2 teaspoons baking powder
¼ cup sugar
1 egg, beaten
1 cup soy milk
2 tablespoons non-dairy margarine, melted
1½ cups whole blueberries (fresh or frozen)

In a bowl, sift together the first three ingredients. Blend the egg, soy milk and margarine, separately, then add to the dry mixture and mix until the large lumps are gone. Fold in the berries. Fill muffin tins 2/3 full; bake in preheated 425° oven for 20-25 minutes.

NUTRIENTS, per muffin:

Calories 139	Protein 3 gm	Carbohydrates 26 gm
Calcium 16 mg	Total fat 3 gm	Saturated fat 0.4 gm

EXCHANGES, not applicable

EGGS & SOUFFLES

Eggs are relatively low calorie, high protein foods. While both the whites and yolks contribute protein, the latter component contains fat and cholesterol; the whites furnish riboflavin. The so-called liquid egg substitutes -- used often in this book -- are derived from egg whites and are essentially free from fat, with no cholesterol; they are best used in cooking recipes and for partial replacement of eggs in omelets and souffles.

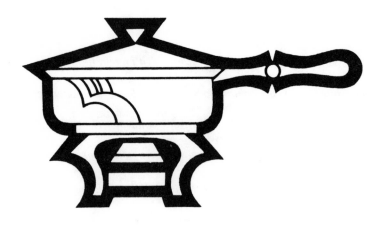

SCRAMBLED EGGS   *4 servings*

6 eggs, at room temperature
1 tablespoon non-dairy margarine
2 tablespoons lactose-reduced milk
pepper to taste

Break the eggs into a small bowl and mix with a fork. Melt the margarine in a skillet, reduce the heat to "low", add the egg mixture and cook with constant stirring until done as desired.

NUTRIENTS, per serving:

Calories 134	Protein 9.5 gm	Carbohydrates 1.3 gm
Calcium 51 mg	Total fat 10 gm	Saturated fat 3 gm

EXCHANGES, per serving: 1½ meat; ½ fat

OMELET SOUFFLE   *4 servings*

¼ cup soy milk
3 egg yolks
¼ cup egg substitute
3 egg whites
1 tablespoon non-dairy margarine

Combine and beat the soy milk, egg yolks and egg substitute. Beat the egg whites separately until stiff; fold into the egg yolk mixture. Pour into the hot, non-stick greased skillet. Cook for 5 minutes, then complete cooking in a 350° oven for an additional 5 minutes. This dish may be served with powdered sugar or a little jam.

NUTRIENTS, per serving:

| Calories 66 | Protein 6 gm | Carbohydrates 0.5 gm |
| Calcium 25 mg | Total fat 4.3 gm | Saturated fat 1.3 gm |

EXCHANGES, per serving: 1 meat

VEGETABLE OMELET   *2 servings*

¼ cup chopped green peppers
1 chopped green onion
4 sliced mushrooms
1 teaspoon oil
1 egg
½ cup egg substitute
pepper to taste

In a non-stick skillet, brown the vegetables in oil until soft; season.
Beat eggs and pour over vegetables, cover and cook until set.

NUTRIENTS, per serving:

| Calories 125 | Protein 15 gm | Carbohydrates 1 gm |
| Calcium 64 mg | Total fat 6 gm | Saturated fat 1.5 gm |

EXCHANGES, per serving: 2 meat

SCRAMBLED EGGS WITH TOFU *4 servings*

1 pound tofu, pressed dry
½ teaspoon minced garlic
2 tablespoons non-dairy margarine
1 egg lightly beaten
½ cup egg substitute
pepper to taste

Mash the tofu. Saute the garlic in the margarine until light brown;
add the tofu, then the beaten egg mixture. Stir; add pepper. Cook
covered over medium heat for 2 minutes; turn and cook for 2 more
minutes (do not overcook).

NUTRIENTS, per serving:

Calories 146	Protein 11 gm	Carbohydrates 1.8 gm
Calcium 99 mg	Total fat 11 gm	Saturated fat 1.8 gm

EXCHANGES, per serving: 1½ meat; ½ fat

SHIRRED EGGS *4 servings*

½ teaspoon non-dairy margarine
4 eggs
4 teaspoons non-dairy cream
1/8 teaspoon paprika

Break each egg carefully into a greased ramekin. Place 1 teaspoon
non-dairy creamer on top of each egg and bake in a 350° oven for 6-8
minutes. Garnish with paprika. Serve with cooked asparagus.

NUTRIENTS, per serving:

Calories 89	Protein 6 gm	Carbohydrates 1 gm
Calcium 38 mg	Total fat 7 gm	Saturated fat 2 gm

EXCHANGES, per serving: 1 meat; ½ fat

EGGS BENEDICT   *6 servings*

6 round slices of milk-free toast
6 slices cooked chicken or turkey breast, 2 ounces each
6 poached eggs (cooked 3-5 minutes in boiling water)
Hollandaise sauce, pg. 78, 1 teaspoon per serving

Place a slice of chicken over each piece of toast; top with a poached egg and cover with 1 tablespoon Hollandaise Sauce.

NUTRIENTS, per serving:

Calories 313	Protein 18 gm	Carbohydrates 13 gm
Calcium 65 mg	Total fat 23 gm	Saturated fat 4 gm

EXCHANGES, per serving: 2½ meat; 1 bread; 2½ fat

ONION MUSHROOM QUICHE   *4 servings*

1 cup cooked brown rice
2 chopped green onions
¼ cup cooked mushrooms
2 eggs
½ cup egg substitute
1½ cups soy milk
pepper to taste
½ cup grated cheddar cheese substitute

Spray 4 small custard dishes (about 4 inch diameter) with cooking spray; press ¼ cup cooked rice into bottom of each dish. Sprinkle each with green onion, mushrooms and cheese substitute. Beat together eggs, milk and pepper and pour into the custard dishes. Bake at 350° for about 20 minutes or until set; serve hot.

NUTRIENTS, per serving:

Calories 206	Protein 16 gm	Carbohydrates 8 gm
Calcium 190 mg	Total fat 13 gm	Saturated fat 6 gm

EXCHANGES, per serving: 2 meat; ½ bread; ½ fat

CARROT SOUFFLE   *6 servings*

4 cups cooked carrots, pureed
2 tablespoons non-dairy margarine
4 tablespoons brown sugar
¼ teaspoons ground nutmeg
½ teaspoon grated lemon peel
4 eggs, separated

To the carrots add the remaining ingredients (except the eggs), mix well and cool slightly. Add the lightly beaten egg yolks to the carrot mixture, mixing gently; let cool slightly. Beat the egg whites until stiff; fold gently into carrot mixture. Bake in 1 quart casserole dish, in preheated 350° oven for about 30 minutes, until set. Serve immediately.

NUTRIENTS, per serving:

Calories 125	Protein 5 gm	Carbohydrates 10 gm
Calcium 36 mg	Total fat 8 gm	Saturated fat 1.5 gm

EXCHANGES, not applicable

SPINACH SOUFFLE 6 servings

1 tablespoon non-dairy margarine
¼ cup finely chopped onions
1 cup chopped frozen spinach, defrosted
2 tablespoons lemon juice
1½ cups white sauce (see section on Sauces & Gravies)
6 eggs, separated
1 egg white

In a non-stick pan, melt the margarine; saute the onions until soft; add the drained spinach and lemon juice and continue to saute for 10 minutes. Set aside. To the prepared white sauce, beat in the egg yolks, one at a time. Stir in the spinach. Beat the egg whites until stiff, then fold into the spinach mixture. Bake in a greased souffle dish, in a preheated 375° oven for 35 minutes. Serve immediately.

NUTRIENTS, per serving:

Calories 150	Protein 8 gm	Carbohydrates 2 gm
Calcium 55 mg	Total fat 13 gm	Saturated fat 2 gm

EXCHANGES, per serving: 1 meat; ½ vegetable; 1½ fat

BROCCOLI SOUFFLE 6 servings

2 tablespoons non-dairy margarine
1½ tablespoons flour
½ cup soy milk
1 tablespoon chopped onion
2 eggs, beaten
¼ cup egg substitute
pepper to taste
2½ cups frozen chopped broccoli, defrosted and drained
¼ cup non-dairy bread crumbs

Melt the margarine; remove from heat and stir in the flour until smooth. Add the milk, onion, eggs and egg substitute, and pepper; blend in the broccoli. Add the broccoli mixture in a greased souffle dish and sprinkle with the bread crumbs. Bake in a 350° oven for 45 minutes, until set.

NUTRIENTS, per serving:

Calories 94	Protein 7 gm	Carbohydrates 6.5 gm
Calcium 6 mg	Total fat 4.5 gm	Saturated fat 0.8 gm

EXCHANGES, per serving: 1 meat; 1 vegetable

CHICKEN SOUFFLE   *4 servings*

4 servings instant mashed potatoes
2 eggs, separated
¼ cup egg substitute
1 cup chopped or coarsely ground cooked chicken
(meat or fish may be substituted)
1 tablespoon minced onions

Prepare 4 servings mashed potatoes according to package directions, using water and milk-free margarine. Cool. Add egg yolks, egg substitute and mashed potatoes; beat well. Add chicken, onion and parsley. Beat egg whites until stiff and fold into chicken mixture. Pour into 1½ quart casserole. Bake 45 minutes in a preheated 350° oven.

NUTRIENTS, per serving:

Calories 188	Protein 18 gm	Carbohydrates 10 gm
Calcium 43 mg	Total fat 9 gm	Saturated fat 2 gm

EXCHANGES, per serving: 2 meat; ½ bread

PANCAKES, CREPES

& FRENCH TOAST

Pancakes and crepes make good bases for meals, since addition of fish, meat, fruit or vegetables afford balanced, tasty dishes.

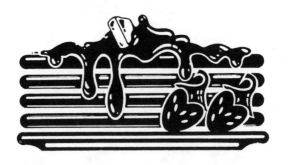

PANCAKES   *4 servings*

1 cup non-dairy pancake mix
1 cup soy milk
1 egg
2 tablespoons vegetable oil

Combine and stir the pancake mix, soy milk and egg until no large lumps remain. Pour ¼ cup of batter onto a greased griddle and cook until golden brown on each side. This recipe makes 8 pancakes; 2 per serving. For variations, add ¼ cup non-dairy chocolate chips to batter before cooking.

NUTRIENTS, per serving:

Calories 197	Protein 6 gm	Carbohydrates 24 gm
Calcium 83 mg	Total fat 9 gm	Saturated fat 1 gm

EXCHANGES, per serving: 1½ bread; 2 fat

APPLE PANCAKES   *4 servings*

2 tablespoons vegetable oil
1 medium Granny Smith apple, peeled and thinly sliced
2 tablespoons sugar
1 teaspoon cinnamon
pancake batter, made according to previous recipe

Saute (in a large skillet) the apple in vegetable oil until soft; add the sugar blended with the cinnamon to the sauteed apples in the skillet. Pour the pancake batter over the fruit. Continue to cook until the underside is brown; turn and cook the other side. Section into quarters and serve.

NUTRIENTS, per serving:

Calories 349	Protein 6 gm	Carbohydrates 37 gm
Calcium 83 mg	Total fat 16 gm	Saturated fat 1 gm

EXCHANGES, not applicable

BUCKWHEAT PANCAKES   *8 servings*

1 package dry yeast
1 tablespoon brown sugar
2 cups buckwheat flour
½ cup corn meal
2½ cups hot water
1 teaspoon baking soda
2 tablespoons vegetable oil

In a bowl, combine all dry ingredients except baking soda. Add hot water. Beat 2 minutes on medium speed. Cover with towel and allow to rise overnight in warm place. In the morning, stir the mixture well. Add baking soda dissolved in 1 teaspoon warm water and oil; mix again. Bake on hot, greased griddle. Serve with syrup. This recipe makes 16 pancakes, 2 per serving.

NUTRIENTS, per serving:

Calories 137	Protein 3 gm	Carbohydrates 21 gm
Calcium 8 mg	Total fat 4 gm	Saturated fat 0.4 gm

EXCHANGES, not applicable

WAFFLES

6 servings

1¾ *cups flour*
3 *teaspoons baking powder*
1/8 *teaspoon cinnamon*
2 *eggs*
2 *egg whites*
½ *cup tofu, mashed*
¾ *cup water*
1 *tablespoon honey*
2 *teaspoons vanilla*
2 *tablespoons non-dairy margarine, melted*

Combine dry ingredients in a bowl. In a separate bowl, place the eggs and egg whites; blend in tofu, water, honey, vanilla and margarine until smooth. Add the liquid to the dry mixture; stir only until thoroughly moistened. Bake in a heated waffle iron until steaming stops and waffle is golden brown. This recipe makes 6 waffles, 1 per serving.

NUTRIENTS, per serving:

Calories 250	Protein 7 gm	Carbohydrates 34 gm
Calcium 31 mg	Total fat 5 gm	Saturated fat 0.5 gm

EXCHANGES, per serving: 2 bread; 1 fat

FRENCH TOAST

4 servings

1 *egg*
2 *tablespoons egg substitute*
½ *cup soy milk*
½ *teaspoon vanilla*
4 *pieces of non-dairy, day old challah, cut into 1 inch slices and trimmed of crust*
2 *tablespoons vegetable oil*
¼ *teaspoon cinnamon*

Beat the eggs with the egg substitutes; add the soy milk and vanilla and beat lightly. Dip each piece of challah in the egg mixture for 2-3 seconds and cook on a lightly greased griddle until brown on each side. Sprinkle with cinnamon before serving.

NUTRIENTS, per serving:

Calories 251	Protein 7.7 gm	Carbohydrates 22 gm
Calcium 75 mg	Total fat 14.3 gm	Saturated fat 2.5 gm

EXCHANGES, per serving: 1½ bread; 3 fat

BAKED FRENCH TOAST   *8 servings*

3 eggs
3 egg whites
1 pound tofu
¼ cup honey
1 teaspoon vanilla
1 teaspoon lemon rind
½ teaspoon nutmeg
¼ cup water
8 pieces non-dairy, day old challah, cut into 1 inch slices and trimmed of crust

In a blender, puree all ingredients, except the bread (add the tofu gradually) until smooth. Line the bottom of a 9 x 13 inch baking dish with the challah. Pour the tofu mixture over the bread. Sprinkle lightly with nutmeg. Bake in a preheated 350° oven for 20 to 30 minutes, until the custard has set. Serve plain or with fresh fruit.

NUTRIENTS, per serving:

Calories 180	Protein 4.6 gm	Carbohydrates 28 gm
Calcium 51 mg	Total fat 5 gm	Saturated fat 1 gm

EXCHANGES, not applicable

CREPES   *6 servings*

3 eggs
½ cup water
1½ cups flour
1 cup water
1 teaspoon non-dairy margarine

Beat eggs with ½ cup water. Add flour and 1 cup water and beat again until thoroughly blended. Heat a greased 5 inch non-stick skillet on low flame. Pour in about 2 tablespoons batter and turn the pan so that the batter spreads over the entire bottom. Cook on one side until the top is dry. Turn onto a paper towel. Continue this process until all the batter has been used.

Fill crepes with chopped vegetables, fruit, creamed chicken, creamed beef or shrimp. A serving is 3 crepes.

NUTRIENTS, per 3 unfilled crepes:

Calories 145	Protein 6 gm	Carbohydrates 22 gm
Calcium 19 mg	Total fat 4 gm	Saturated fat 1 gm

EXCHANGES, per serving: ½ meat; 1½ bread

SAUCES & DRESSINGS

Sauces and dressings improve the taste and eye appeal of many dishes. With small changes in ingredients, countless variations are possible. While the basic sauces for meat, eggs, fish and vegetables are WHITE, BROWN and EGG-based, the list goes on to include peanut sauce and chocolate sauce.

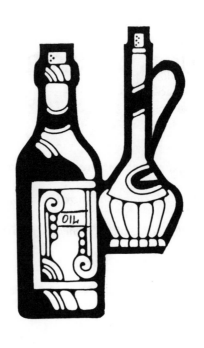

WHITE SAUCE I

1 cup

2 tablespoons non-dairy margarine
2 tablespoons flour
1 cup lactose-reduced milk
1 teaspoon dry sherry
2 tablespoons chopped chives

Melt margarine in small saucepan; remove from heat, add flour and stir until smooth. Add the milk substitute gradually over low heat and stir until thick. Add sherry. Use in souffles; add pepper and use over fish fillets and chicken; addition of 2 tablespoons of shredded, sauteed lobster meat converts this dish into Newburg sauce, to be used over baked fish fillets; and this sauce is excellent over poached eggs and asparagus.

<u>NUTRIENTS</u>, per tablespoon:

Calories 23	Protein 0.6 gm	Carbohydrates 1 gm
Calcium 19 mg	Total fat 1.8 gm	Saturated fat 0.3 gm

<u>EXCHANGES</u>, per tablespoon: free

WHITE SAUCE II

1 cup

3 tablespoons non-dairy margarine
3 tablespoons flour
1 cup chicken bouillon
1/8 teaspoon finely chopped onion
pepper to taste
1/8 teaspoon basil

Melt margarine in a small saucepan. Add flour and stir over low heat until mixture is smooth. Gradually stir in bouillon, stirring constantly, until mixture is thick. Add onion, pepper and basil. Serve with vegetables, over eggs or over shredded chicken.

NUTRIENTS, per tablespoon:

Calories 26	Protein 0.4 gm	Carbohydrates 1 gm
Calcium 1.5 mg	Total fat 2 gm	Saturated fat 0.4 gm

EXCHANGES, per tablespoon: ½ fat

QUICK WHITE SAUCES   *1 cup*
(for fish dishes)

2 tablespoons non-dairy margarine
2 tablespoons flour
1 cup soy milk
pepper to taste
1 tablespoon white wine

In a small saucepan, blend margarine and flour together until smooth; add the soy milk, a little at a time, while stirring. Heat to boiling, stirring constantly and cook for a minute or two. Add pepper. If used, add the wine. This basic sauce permits you to make a variety of white sauces quickly; all go well with fish.

Anchovy sauce: to one cup basic sauce add 1 teaspoon chopped canned anchovies.

Cheese sauce: to one cup basic sauce add 1 tablespoon grated hard (Swiss, Parmesan or Cheddar) cheese, if tolerated.

Egg sauce: to one cup basic sauce add 1 hard cooked egg, finely chopped.

Horseradish sauce: to one cup basic sauce add 1 tablespoon grated horseradish.

Shrimp sauce: to one cup basic sauce add two tablespoons finely chopped cooked shrimp.

Mustard sauce: to one cup of basic sauce, add 1 teaspoon dry mustard.

Lime sauce: to one cup of basic sauce, add 1 tablespoon lime juice.

Turmeric sauce: to one cup of the basic sauce, add 1 tablespoon tumeric powder.

NUTRIENTS, per tablespoon of basic sauce:

Calories 20	Protein 0.6 gm	Carbohydrates 0.8 gm
Calcium 19 mg	Total fat 1.7 gm	Saturated fat 0.3 gm

EXCHANGES, per tablespoon: free

WHITE SAUCE BASE   *1 cup*

1 tablespoon non-dairy margarine
¾ teaspoon flour
1 cup soy milk
¼ teaspoon crushed garlic

Blend margarine and flour in a saucepan; heat and stir for 3 minutes. Add the soy milk gradually, then the garlic; simmer for 5 minutes. While this sauce may be used as is on vegetables or seafood, it serves as a base for a variety of sauces:

Sauce Florentine: to 1 cup of the base, add 1 cup finely chopped spinach; simmer for 2-3 minutes. Use over eggs and fish.

Sauce Italian: to 1 cup of the base, add ½ tablespoon olive oil, ½teaspoon finely chopped red or green pepper and ½ teaspoon oregano; simmer for 5 minutes. Serve over salad.

NUTRIENTS, per tablespoon of basic sauce:

Calories 30	Protein 3 gm	Carbohydrates 2 gm
Calcium 75 mg	Total fat 1.6 gm	Saturated fat 0.4 gm

EXCHANGES, per tablespoon: free

HORSERADISH SAUCE I   *2 cups*

2 cups non-dairy (whippable) cream or
3 cups non-dairy whipped topping
1 teaspoon lemon juice
¼ cup white horseradish, drained
pepper to taste

Whip the non-dairy cream (or start with the whipped topping), then add the sugar, a bit at a time. Add the lemon juice, horseradish and the pepper, mixing well. Keep cold; serve with fish or meat.

NUTRIENTS, per tablespoon:

Calories 19	Protein 0 gm	Carbohydrates 2 gm
Calcium 0 mg	Total fat 2 gm	Saturated fat 0.5 gm

EXCHANGES, not applicable

HORSERADISH SAUCE II   *1 cup*

1 cup mayonnaise
¼ cup (drained) white horseradish
½ cup non-pasteurized yogurt
pepper to taste

Blend all ingredients; serve with smoked fish.

NUTRIENTS, per tablespoon:

Calories 104	Protein 0.6 gm	Carbohydrates 0.9 gm
Calcium 14 mg	Total fat 11 gm	Saturated fat 2 gm

EXCHANGES, per tablespoon: 2 fat

SAUCE A LA KING   *1 cup*

½ cup chopped fresh mushrooms
1 tablespoon chopped green pepper
2 tablespoons non-dairy margarine
1 ½ tablespoons flour
1/8 teaspoon white pepper
½ cup non-dairy cream
½ cup chicken bouillon

Saute mushrooms and pepper in the margarine over low heat until soft; add 3-4 tablespoons of the liquid (non-dairy creamer or chicken soup), stir in the flour. When blended, add the remaining liquid; heat but do not boil. Blend with tuna, salmon, chicken or diced meat; season, and serve over toast, rice or use to fill crepes. Note: If made with chicken soup, the caloric content is reduced by 50% and the fat content by 75%.

NUTRIENTS, per tablespoon:

Calories 16	Protein 1.0 gm	Carbohydrates 1.5 gm
Calcium 0.6 mg	Total fat 1.4 gm	Saturated fat 0.1 gm

EXCHANGES, per tablespoon: free

CREAMY DILL SAUCE   *1 cup*

1 tablespoon cornstarch
1 cup chicken bouillon
½ teaspoon dried dill
½ cup non-pasteurized yogurt

Blend cornstarch with small amount of bouillon; add remaining
bouillon and bring to boil. Add dill and yogurt. Use with meat or
vegetables.

NUTRIENTS, per tablespoon:

Calories 11	Protein 1.7 gm	Carbohydrates 1.6 gm
Calcium 13 mg	Total fat 0.2 gm	Saturated fat 1.1 gm

EXCHANGES, per tablespoon: free

CUSTARD SAUCE   *2 cups*

2 tablespoons cornstarch
1 cup non-dairy cream
1 cup lactose-reduced milk
¼ cup sugar
¼ teaspoon grated orange peel
1 teaspoon vanilla

Blend the cornstarch with ¼ cup of the cream until smooth. Set aside.
Combine the remaining cream with the rest of the ingredients in a
saucepan and bring to a boil with stirring. Add the cornstarch base,
stir gently, and cook until the sauce begins to thicken. Serve over
warm fruit desserts.

NUTRIENTS, per tablespoon:

Calories 43	Protein 0 gm	Carbohydrates 7 gm
Calcium 19 mg	Total fat 2 gm	Saturated fat 0 gm

EXCHANGES, not applicable

FRUIT TOPPING   *1 cup*

1 cup apricot nectar
2 tablespoons sugar
1 tablespoon cornstarch
2 tablespoons cold water

Heat the nectar and sugar to boiling. Mix cornstarch with cold water to a smooth paste. Add to hot nectar, stirring constantly. Cook slowly until thick and clear. Serve with pudding, desserts or cereals.

NUTRIENTS, per tablespoon:

Calories 9	Protein 0 gm	Carbohydrates 2 mg
Calcium 1 mg	Total fat 0 gm	Saturated fat 0 gm

EXCHANGES, not applicable

MOCK SOUR CREAM I   *1 cup*

8 ounces low-lactose cottage cheese
1 tablespoon cider vinegar
1 teaspoon non-dairy cream

Blend all ingredients in a blender until the consistency of sour cream.

NUTRIENTS, per tablespoon:

Calories 18	Protein 3 gm	Carbohydrates 0.3 gm
Calcium 14 mg	Total fat 0.3 gm	Saturated fat 0.2 gm

EXCHANGES, per tablespoon: free

MOCK SOUR CREAM II   *1 cup*

1 cup non-pasteurized yogurt
1 teaspoon lemon juice
1 teaspoon vegetable oil

Blend ingredients gently with a spoon until completely smooth and creamy. For different flavor, add ¼ cup chives.

NUTRIENTS, per tablespoon:

Calories 11	Protein 0.8 gm	Carbohydrates 1 gm
Calcium 25 mg	Total fat 0.5 gm	Saturated fat 0.2 gm

EXCHANGES, per tablespoon: free

MOCK YOGURT   *2 cups*

10 ounces sweetened canned pineapple chunks
2 tablespoons syrup from pineapple chunks
1 teaspoons vanilla extract
5 ounces tofu

Blend all the ingredients in a blender until the consistency of yogurt, 15-30 seconds. Other fruits, including raspberries, strawberries and bananas can be used in place of pineapple to flavor this sauce. Eat as is, or serve cold over fruit.

<u>NUTRIENTS</u>, per tablespoon:

Calories 12	Protein 0.5 gm	Carbohydrates 2 gm
Calcium 9 mg	Total fat 0.3 gm	Saturated fat 0.1 gm

<u>EXCHANGES</u>, not applicable

MOCK COTTAGE CHEESE   *6 servings*

16 ounces tofu
2 tablespoons vegetable oil
pepper or cinnamon to taste

Using a fork, mash the tofu until the consistency of cottage cheese;
blend in the oil and spice. Serve either variety over hot, cooked
noodles or use the peppered version when making lasagna.

<u>NUTRIENTS</u>, per serving:

Calories 88	Protein 5.2 gm	Carbohydrates 1.6 gm
Calcium 87 mg	Total fat 7 gm	Saturated fat 1 gm

<u>EXCHANGES</u>, per serving: 1 meat; ½ fat

BROWN SAUCE   *2 cups*

2 tablespoons non-dairy margarine
3 tablespoons flour
2 cups beef bouillon
pepper to taste

Melt the margarine over low heat; stir in the flour and continue stirring and cooking for 2 minutes. Gradually add the bouillon and pepper; cook until smooth. Use over beef or mashed potatoes. For variety, the following may be added to 2 cups of sauce: ¼ cup chopped sauteed mushrooms; 2 tablespoons minced sauteed onions; or 2 tablespoons prepared mustard.

NUTRIENTS, per tablespoon:

Calories 10	Protein 0.2 gm	Carbohydrates 0.7 gm
Calcium 0.7 mg	Total fat 0.8 gm	Saturated fat 0.2 gm

EXCHANGES, per tablespoon: free

SAUCE STROGANOFF   *2 cups*

2 cups beef bouillon
2 tablespoons flour
¼ cup tomato sauce
½ tablespoon Worcestshire sauce
2 tablespoons mayonnaise
¼ teaspoon paprika
½ cup mock sour cream

Pour the beef bouillon in a saucepan, add the flour and blend well. Add the tomato sauce and Worcestershire sauce; then cook until smooth and thick, stirring constantly to prevent lumps. Remove from the heat; stir in the mayonnaise and paprika. Just before using, stir in sour cream. Use the sauce over hot braised beef, broiled lamb chops, or grilled or stewed chicken.

NUTRIENTS, per ½ cup

Calories 82	Protein 1 gm	Carbohydrates 4 gm
Calcium 4 mg	Total fat 7 gm	Saturated fat 1.5 gm

EXCHANGES, per ½ cup: 1½ fat

HUNTER'S SAUCE   *2 cups*

3 tablespoons non-dairy marg.   e
1 tablespoon finely chopped onions
1 cup finely chopped mushrooms
½ cup dry white wine
¼ cup tomato paste
1 cup chicken bouillon
1 teaspoon chopped parsley

Melt the margarine in a pan, saute the onions until soft and transparent; add the mushrooms and continue to saute for 3-4 minutes. Add the wine and heat until the liquid volume is reduced by half. Add the tomato paste, bouillon and chopped parsley; cook for 2-3 minutes with stirring. Serve hot over sauteed or broiled chicken.

NUTRIENTS, per tablespoon:

Calories 16	Protein 0.1 gm	Carbohydrates 0.9 gm
Calcium 1 mg	Total fat 1 gm	Saturated fat 0.2 gm

EXCHANGES, per tablespoon: free

HOLLANDAISE SAUCE   *1 cup*

2 egg yolks
¼ cup egg substitute
¾ cup hot water
1 tablespoon lemon juice
½ cup non-dairy margarine, melted
white pepper to taste

Beat egg mixture in saucepan, over very low heat until it begins to thicken; continue to heat, adding the hot water gradually. Add lemon juice. Slowly pour hot margarine into egg mixture, beating until fluffy. Add pepper and serve hot over vegetables.

NUTRIENTS, per tablespoon:

Calories 60	Protein 0.8 gm	Carbohydrates 0.1 gm
Calcium 5 mg	Total fat 6 gm	Saturated fat 1.3 gm

EXCHANGES, per tablespoon: 1 fat

Note: Many variations of Hollandaise Sauce are possible. For example, to 1 cup of sauce add one of the following: 3 tablespoons non-dairy whipped topping, 3 tablespoons drained, chopped fresh cucumber, 2 tablespoons dry white wine. These modified versions may be used over vegetables or eggs.

EGG FREE HOLLANDAISE SAUCE   *1 cup*

1 cup soy milk
2 tablespoons vegetable oil
1 tablespoon cornstarch blended in 2 tablespoons water
1 tablespoon lemon juice
⅛ teaspoon paprika

Combine the first 3 ingredients in a saucepan and simmer for 3 minutes, stirring constantly. When mixture is thick, add lemon juice. Serve hot, over vegetables, garnished with paprika.

NUTRIENTS, per tablespoon:

Calories 17	Protein 0.3 gm	Carbohydrates 0.1 gm
Calcium 11 mg	Total fat 2 gm	Saturated fat 0.2 gm

EXCHANGES, per tablespoon: ½ fat

MAYONNAISE I
1¾ cups

1 egg
2 egg whites
1 teaspoon sugar
1¼ cups salad oil
2 tablespoons lemon juice
1 tablespoon vinegar

Place egg and egg whites, sugar and one-quarter cup oil in blender and blend thoroughly. While blender is running, remove cover and add one-half cup oil, lemon juice, and vinegar and blend; slowly add the remaining oil and blend until thick.

NUTRIENTS, per tablespoon:

Calories 90	Protein 0.5 gm	Carbohydrates 0.04 gm
Calcium 1.3 mg	Total fat 10 gm	Saturated fat 1 gm

EXCHANGES, per tablespoon: 2 fat

MAYONNAISE II
1½ cups

1 cup soy milk
½ cup olive oil
2 teaspoons vinegar
1 teaspoon honey
¼ teaspoon dried mustard

Pour the soy milk into a blender. While at low speed, slowly add the remaining ingredients and blend until the mixture is creamy; chill before serving.

NUTRIENTS, per tablespoon:

Calories 43	Protein 0.2 gm	Carbohydrates 0.8 gm
Calcium 5 mg	Total fat 4.6 gm	Saturated fat 0.6 gm

EXCHANGES, per tablespoon: 1 fat

GREEN GODDESS DRESSING   *2 cups*

2 cups mayonnaise
½ teaspoon crushed garlic
2 tablespoons chives, chopped
1 tablespoon parsley flakes
3 anchovy fillets
1 tablespoon vinegar
2 teaspoons lemon juice
½ cup non-pasteurized yogurt

Blend ingredients until smooth. Refrigerate. Serve with fish or shellfish.

NUTRIENTS, per tablespoon:

Calories 102	Protein 0.4 gm	Carbohydrates 0.7 gm
Calcium 8 mg	Total fat 11 gm	Saturated fat 1.7 gm

EXCHANGES, per tablespoon: 2 fat

TARTAR SAUCE   *1 cup*

1 cup mayonnaise
½ cup chopped dill pickle
2 tablespoons cider vinegar
⅛ teaspoon onion powder

Combine all ingredients in a bowl, and stir until smooth. Serve with fish.

NUTRIENTS, per tablespoon:

Calories 100	Protein 0.2 gm	Carbohydrates 0.4 gm
Calcium 2 mg	Total fat 11 gm	Saturated fat 1.6 gm

EXCHANGES, per tablespoon: 2 fat

LEMON-VINEGAR DRESSING   *1 cup*

¾ cup olive oil
2 teaspoons grated lemon rind
2 teaspoons dry mustard
pepper to taste
2 tablespoons lemon juice

Blend the first four ingredients, then add the lemon juice. Serve over bean salads.

NUTRIENTS, per tablespoon:

Calories 90	Protein 0 gm	Carbohydrates 0 gm
Calcium 0 mg	Total fat 10 gm	Saturated fat 1.4 gm

EXCHANGES, per tablespoon: 2 fat

HERB DRESSING   *1 cup*

3 tablespoons lemon juice
1 tablespoon vegetable oil
2 tablespoons water
1 clove garlic, minced
½ teaspoon powdered ginger
⅛ teaspoon celery seed
pepper to taste
¼ cup chopped parsley
½ cup tofu, mashed

In a blender, combine all ingredients except tofu. With blender running, add tofu, a little at a time, and blend until dressing is thick and smooth, about 1 minute.

NUTRIENTS, per tablespoon:

Calories 10	Protein 0.3 gm	Carbohydrates 0.1 gm
Calcium 4 mg	Total fat 1 gm	Saturated fat 0.2 gm

EXCHANGES, per tablespoon: free

RUSSIAN DRESSING   *1 cup*

3½ tablespoons tomato catsup
¼ cup water
2 tablespoons lemon juice
2 tablespoons olive oil
1 teaspoon Worcestershire sauce
2 ounces tofu

Combine all ingredients but the tofu in a blender. With the blender on, add the tofu in small pieces; blend until creamy.

NUTRIENTS, per tablespoon:

Calories 20	Protein 0.2 gm	Carbohydrates 0.9 gm
Calcium 2.7 mg	Total fat 1.8 gm	Saturated fat 0.3 gm

EXCHANGES, per tablespoon: free

LEMON CREAM DRESSING   *½ cup*

¼ cup vegetable oil
2 tablespoons soy milk
1 tablespoon lemon juice
½ teaspoon honey
8 ounces tofu

In a blender, combine all ingredients except the tofu; add the tofu in small pieces to the other ingredients. Blend until smooth. Chill. Use in place of sour cream with potatoes or soup.

NUTRIENTS, per tablespoon:

Calories 74	Protein 1 gm	Carbohydrates 1.5 gm
Calcium 20 mg	Total fat 7 gm	Saturated fat 0.8 gm

EXCHANGES, per tablespoon: 1½ fat

HONEY LIME DRESSING   *1 cup*

¾ cup French dressing
2 tablespoons honey
2 tablespoons lime juice
½ teaspoon dried dill weed, chopped

Combine ingredients in covered jar; shake vigorously. Chill well before serving over fruit such as melon or sliced peaches.

NUTRIENTS, per tablespoon:

Calories 75	Protein 0.1 gm	Carbohydrates 8 gm
Calcium 1.6 mg	Total fat 5 gm	Saturated fat 1 gm

EXCHANGES, not applicable

PEANUT SAUCE   *½ cup*

1 tablespoon sesame oil
½ cup sesame seeds
2 tablespoons soy sauce
½ teaspoon chili oil
1 teaspoon honey
1 tablespoon wine vinegar
½ teaspoon minced garlic
1 tablespoon vegetable oil
1 tablespoon creamy peanut butter

In a skillet containing the sesame oil, brown the sesame seeds; remove from heat. Add the remaining ingredients to the skillet; blend well. Serve cold over cooked, cold pasta or warm over heated chicken or turkey.

NUTRIENTS, per tablespoon:

Calories 126	Protein 3.6 gm	Carbohydrates 5 gm
Calcium 13 mg	Total fat 11 gm	Saturated fat 1 gm

EXCHANGES, not applicable

CHOCOLATE SAUCE

1 cup

1/3 cup bittersweet chocolate chips
½ cup sugar
½ cup non-dairy cream, warmed
1 tablespoon rum
3 tablespoons water
¼ teaspoon vanilla

Blend all ingredients in an electric blender until smooth. Serve over non-dairy ice cream or pudding.

<u>NUTRIENTS</u>, per tablespoon:

Calories 46	Protein 0.2 gm	Carbohydrates 8 gm
Calcium 8.5 mg	Total fat 1.6 gm	Saturated fat 0.8 gm

<u>EXCHANGES</u>, not applicable

VEGETABLES & PASTA

All vegetables are cholesterol-free, with very little fat; carrots are high in vitamin A; kale is high is calcium; pasta furnishes carbohydrates and the B-vitamins.

And some lentil-based dishes are flavorful substitutes for meat in recipes such as mock chopped liver.

FIVE BEAN SALAD   *6 servings*

½ cup of each of the following canned beans:
whole green
wax
kidney
cannelini
garbanzo

½ cup sugar
1 cup wine vinegar
1 medium onion, thinly sliced
2 tablespoons olive oil

Drain all the beans, combine in large bowl and set aside. Heat the sugar and vinegar together, then add to the beans mixture. Add the onion and oil; toss. Refrigerate for 6 hours before serving.

NUTRIENTS, per serving:

Calories 184	Protein 4.5 gm	Carbohydrates 31 gm
Calcium 33 mg	Total fat 5 gm	Saturated fat 0.7 gm

EXCHANGES, not applicable

MOCK CHOPPED LIVER I   *4 servings*
(String Bean Pate)

4 cups string beans, cut into 1 inch lengths
1 small onion
2 hard cooked eggs
pepper to taste
chopped garlic to taste
1 tablespoon ground walnuts

Cook the beans and onion in about ½ cup water until soft, about 10 minutes. Mash together with the eggs, spices, and nuts, blending well to the consistency of pate. Serve on crackers.

NUTRIENTS, per serving:

Calories 131	Protein 7.3 gm	Carbohydrates 12 gm
Calcium 80 mg	Total fat 7 gm	Saturated fat 1 gm

EXCHANGES, per serving: 2 vegetable; ½ meat; 1 fat

MOCK CHOPPED LIVER II   *4 servings*
(Lentil Salad)

1 cup lentils, cooked and mashed
1 medium onion, chopped finely
1 hard cooked egg, mashed
2 tablespoons olive oil
garlic powder to taste
pepper to taste

In a non-stick skillet, saute the onions in a little olive oil. In a blender, place the egg, spices and remaining olive oil; add the onions and blend until the mixture is the consistency of pate. Serve cold on crackers.

NUTRIENTS, per serving:

Calories 128	Protein 4.5 gm	Carbohydrates 8.5 gm
Calcium 17 mg	Total fat 10 gm	Saturated fat 2 gm

EXCHANGES, per serving: ½ bread; 2 fat

VEGETABLE BURGERS

6 servings

2 cups canned kidney beans
¼ cup sunflower seeds
1 medium onion, chopped
pepper to taste
2 tablespoons olive oil
¼ cup tomato sauce
½ cup oat bran

Combine the first four ingredients in a blender; blend until smooth. Add the remaining ingredients; mix well. Form into 6 patties and place on a lightly greased cookie sheet. Bake in a 350° oven until browned, about 15 minutes.

NUTRIENTS, per serving:

Calories 226	Protein 9 gm	Carbohydrates 25 gm
Calcium 54 mg	Total fat 11 gm	Saturated fat 1 gm

EXCHANGES, per serving: 1 meat; 1½ bread; 1 fat

BEAN ENCHILADAS

6 servings

1 tablespoon vegetable oil
1 small onion, chopped fine
¾ teaspoon chopped garlic
12 ounces canned pinto beans
4 ounces canned kernel corn, drained
1½ cups tomato sauce
1 teaspoon chili powder
6 corn tortillas
¼ cup non-dairy cheddar cheese, shredded

Heat vegetable oil in a skillet; add onion and garlic and saute for 2 minutes. Add the beans, corn, tomato sauce and seasoning. Cook for 20 minutes. Spoon filling into tortillas; sprinkle each serving with 2 teaspoon cheese. Place under broiler for 1 minute before serving.

NUTRIENTS, per serving:

Calories 300	Protein 15 gm	Carbohydrates 48 gm
Calcium 260 mg	Total fat 7.5 gm	Saturated fat 2 gm

EXCHANGES, per serving: 1 meat; 3 bread; ½ fat

CREAMED BROCCOLI   *4 servings*

1 10 ounce package frozen chopped broccoli, cooked & drained
1 can (about 1¼ cups) non-dairy mushroom soup
¼ cup soy milk
¼ cup mayonnaise
1 egg, beaten

Place the broccoli in a 1½ quart lightly greased casserole dish. Cover with the sauce obtained by blending the remaining ingredients. Cover and bake in a preheated 350° oven for 30 minutes.

NUTRIENTS, per serving:

Calories 180	Protein 5 gm	Carbohydrates 7 gm
Calcium 118 mg	Total fat 12 gm	Saturated fat 2.9 gm

EXCHANGES, per serving: ½ meat; ½ bread; 2 fat

CREAMED ARTICHOKE HEARTS   *4 servings*

1 pound canned marinated artichoke hearts, drained
¼ cup dill sauce (pg. 72)
1 teaspoon grated onion
¼ cup non-dairy bread crumbs

Place vegetable in pan coated with non-stick spray. Blend the cream sauce and onion; add to artichokes. Sprinkle with bread crumbs and bake in a 1 quart (sprayed) casserole dish at 300° for 15 minutes.

NUTRIENTS, per serving:

Calories 100	Protein 3 gm	Carbohydrates 13 gm
Calcium 27 mg	Total fat 1.4 gm	Saturated fat 0.3 gm

EXCHANGES, per serving: ½ bread; 1 vegetable

SPAGHETTI SQUASH   *4 servings*

2 medium sized spaghetti squashes
1 tablespoon non-dairy margarine
8 ounces of canned tomato sauce
1/8 teaspoon oregano

Halve the squashes, dot with margarine and bake at 350° for about 40 minutes, until soft. Meanwhile heat the tomato sauce and oregano until bubbly; pour it over the hot squash. Eat by scoring the squash with a fork, at which time the squash separates into spaghetti-like strands.

NUTRIENTS, per serving:

Calories 109	Protein 2 gm	Carbohydrates 13 gm
Calcium 33 mg	Total fat 5 gm	Saturated fat 0.6 gm

EXCHANGES, per serving: 1 bread; 1 fat

CARROT PUDDING   *6 servings*

3 eggs, separated
3 tablespoons sugar
¼ cup orange juice
1 teaspoon grated orange rind
3 cups shredded raw carrots

Beat egg yolks with sugar until light and fluffy. Gradually add orange juice. Stir in orange rind and carrots. Beat egg whites until stiff but not dry; fold into carrot batter. Turn into a greased 1½ quart casserole. Bake in a 350° oven for 30 minutes.

NUTRIENTS, per serving:

Calories 88	Protein 3.7 gm	Carbohydrates 12 gm
Calcium 29 mg	Total fat 2.8 gm	Saturated fat 0.9 gm

EXCHANGES, not applicable

CREAMED SPINACH   *6 servings*

1 tablespoon non-dairy margarine
1 tablespoon potato starch
2 tablespoons cold water
¾ cup chicken bouillon
pepper to taste
2 ten ounce packages frozen chopped spinach, cooked

Melt the margarine in a saucepan. Dissolve the starch in the water; add this liquid to the margarine, while stirring. Add the bouillon and cook; continue stirring until thick and smooth. Season. Blend the sauce with the spinach and serve hot.

NUTRIENTS, per serving:

Calories 50	Protein 3.5 gm	Carbohydrates 6 gm
Calcium 118 mg	Total fat 2.4 gm	Saturated fat 0.4 gm

EXCHANGES, per serving: 1 vegetable; ½ fat

SPINACH PIE WITH COTTAGE CHEESE   *8 servings*

¼ cup vegetable oil
1½ cups chopped onions
2 ten ounce packages frozen chopped spinach
2 eggs
½ cup liquid egg substitute
½ cup chopped scallions
1 pound low lactose cottage cheese (or 1 pound mashed tofu)
tablespoons dried dill
2 tablespoons dried parsley
pepper to taste
8 ounce (½ package filo leaves)

Heat the oil in a skillet. Saute the onions until brown; add the thawed spinach and continue to saute for 3-4 minutes. Set aside. In a separate bowl, mix the remaining ingredients (except the filo leaves). Add the spinach and onions; blend well.

In a greased 12 inch pan, add 12 leaves of the filo dough, one sheet at a time, fitting each sheet to the pan and oiling each sheet lightly after it has been placed in the pan. Fill with the spinach filling and repeat the process with 12 additional sheets. Oil the top sheet also; with a sharp knife, score the top layer into 8 squares. Bake at 350° for about 70 minutes, until brown. Serve hot.

NUTRIENTS, per serving:

| Calories 250 | Protein 16 gm | Carbohydrates 28 gm |
| Calcium 129 mg | Total fat 8.6 gm | Saturated fat 1.5 gm |

EXCHANGES, per serving: 1½ meat; 1 bread

POTATO PANCAKES   *4 servings*

2 eggs
2 cups grated, raw, unpeeled potatoes
¼ teaspoon baking powder
1 small onion, minced
1 tablespoon potato starch
garlic powder, to taste
pepper, to taste

Beat eggs and mix with potatoes; add remaining ingredients and beat together. Drop by spoonfuls on a hot, oiled griddle. Turn and brown on both sides; drain on absorbent paper. Serve hot with applesauce (this recipe makes 12 pancakes, 3 per serving).

NUTRIENTS, per serving:

| Calories 126 | Protein 4 gm | Carbohydrates 12 gm |
| Calcium 20 mg | Total fat 8 gm | Saturated fat 2 gm |

EXCHANGES, per serving: ½ meat; ¼ bread; 1 fat

BAKED ACORN SQUASH   *6 servings*

3 medium size acorn squashes
1 tablespoon non-dairy margarine
½ cup honey
¼ cup crushed walnuts

Split the squash and remove seeds; brush cavities with melted margarine; add 1 tablespoon honey to each half. Bake in a preheated 350° oven for 50 minutes.

NUTRIENTS, per serving:

Calories 158	Protein 3 gm	Carbohydrates 34 gm
Calcium 21 mg	Total fat 8 gm	Saturated fat 0.7 gm

EXCHANGES, not applicable

ASPARAGUS ON TOAST POINTS *6 servings*

2 teaspoons non-dairy margarine
2 pounds fresh asparagus, washed and trimmed to 2 inch lengths
pepper to taste
3 tablespoons non-dairy cream
6 slices non-dairy white bread, toasted and cut diagonally

Melt the margarine in a small pan; add the asparagus and mix to coat; cook for 3 minutes. Add the pepper and the cream; pour over the asparagus. Serve on the toast.

NUTRIENTS, per serving:

Calories 105	Protein 4 gm	Carbohydrates 17 gm
Calcium 54 mg	Total fat 3 gm	Saturated fat 0.8 gm

EXCHANGES, per serving: 1 bread; ½ fat

STEAMED COLLARDS, KALE, BEET GREENS AND TURNIP GREENS   *3 servings*

½ pound raw collards, kale, beet greens or turnip greens
pepper to taste
1 teaspoon lemon juice

Strip the leaves from the stems; remove tough stems. Wash well.
Cook just barely covered with water for at least 30 minutes. Season
with pepper and/or lemon juice. Serve with meat or potatoes.

NUTRIENTS, per serving:

Calories 22	Protein 2 gm	Carbohydrates 4 gm
Calcium 116 mg	Total fat 0 gm	Saturated fat 0 gm

EXCHANGES, per serving: 1 vegetable

COLLARDS WITH ONIONS AND SPICES   *6 servings*

1 teaspoon non-dairy margarine
¼ cup minced onions
1 pound collard greens, cooked (see previous recipe)
¼ cup chopped mushrooms
¼ teaspoon ginger

Melt the margarine in a non-stick skillet and add the onions; saute
until brown. Add the collard greens and mushrooms; saute for 3-4
minutes, then add the spice. Serve warm with potatoes, meat or
mixed with spinach.

NUTRIENTS, per serving:

Calories 32	Protein 2.3 gm	Carbohydrates 4.6 gm
Calcium 119 mg	Total fat 0.7 gm	Saturated fat 0.1 gm

EXCHANGES, per serving: 1 vegetable

SAUTEED TURNIP GREENS   *6 servings*

1 tablespoon non-dairy margarine
1 pound turnip greens, washed and chopped into ½ inch pieces
½ teaspoon lemon juice

Melt the margarine in a non-stick skillet. Use a paper towel to remove excess moisture from the greens; add to the hot margarine. Saute for about 5 minutes. Blend with lemon juice before serving.

NUTRIENTS, per serving:

Calories 30	Protein 2.2 gm	Carbohydrates 4.4 gm
Calcium 118 mg	Total fat 0.7 gm	Saturated fat 0.1 gm

EXCHANGES, per serving: 1 vegetable

TURNIP SOUFFLE   *6 servings*

6 medium size turnips
1 tablespoon non-dairy margarine
2 tablespoons flour
¼ cup soy milk
2 egg yolks
2 egg whites, beaten stiff

Peel and slice the turnips; cover with water; simmer until tender, about 20 minutes. Drain. Melt the margarine in a small pan, blend in the flour until smooth; add the soy milk and egg yolks; fold in the beaten egg whites. Place the mixture in a greased casserole dish and bake at 375° until done, about 40 minutes.

NUTRIENTS, per serving:

Calories 61	Protein 2.7 gm	Carbohydrates 4 gm
Calcium 28 mg	Total fat 5 gm	Saturated fat 0.8 gm

EXCHANGES, per serving: 1 vegetable, 1 fat

BEANS WITH TORTILLAS   *4 servings*

8 tortillas
1 cup cooked kidney beans
1 tablespoon soy sauce
1 teaspoon chili powder
1 tablespoon vinegar
2 tablespoons non-dairy margarine
½ cup chopped green pepper
½ cup chopped onions
1 cup non-dairy or mock sour cream
1 cup chopped cucumber

Wrap the tortillas in foil and heat at 350° for 5 minutes. Mix the beans, soy sauce, chili powder and vinegar; let stand for 10 minutes. Melt the margarine in a saucepan and saute the pepper and onions until the onions start to brown. Add the bean mixture and heat for another 5 minutes. Fill the tortillas with the bean mixture; top with the sour cream and chopped cucumber. Two tortillas make a serving.

NUTRIENTS, per serving:

Calories 282	Protein 10 gm	Carbohydrates 36.5 gm
Calcium 171 mg	Total fat 11 gm	Saturated fat 2 gm

EXCHANGES, per serving: 1 meat; 2 bread; 1 fat

PASTA WITH CHICKPEAS   8 servings

1 tablespoon non-dairy margarine
1 medium onion, diced
1 medium pepper, diced
2 cups canned chickpeas
1 pound macaroni, cooked according to package directions

In a non-stick skillet, melt the margarine; add the onion and pepper
and saute for 3 minutes. Add the chickpeas and continue heating for
1 minute. Add the cooked macaroni, toss, and serve hot.

NUTRIENTS, per serving:

Calories 200	Protein 7 gm	Carbohydrates 36 gm
Calcium 31 mg	Total fat 2.6 gm	Saturated fat 0.3 gm

EXCHANGES, per serving: 2 bread; 1 vegetable; ½ fat

PASTA PRIMAVERA   4 servings

2 tablespoons olive oil
1 cup cooked broccoli, cut into 1 inch pieces
½ teaspoon minced garlic
1 tablespoon basil
½ teaspoon oregano
pepper to taste
8 ounces spaghetti, cooked according to package directions and drained

In a skillet, heat the olive oil; saute the broccoli for 3-4 minutes; add the seasonings and toss. Add the pasta; toss and serve.

NUTRIENTS, per serving:

Calories 280	Protein 9 gm	Carbohydrates 43 gm
Calcium 60.5 mg	Total fat 7.5 gm	Saturated fat 1.0 gm

EXCHANGES, per serving: 3 bread; 1½ fat

SPAGHETTI WITH HONEY AND SESAME SEEDS   *6 servings*

½ cup soy milk
¼ cup honey
¼ cup sesame (or poppy) seeds
4 cups cooked thin spaghetti, drained

Heat the first three ingredients together in a saucepan for 2-3 minutes; add the noodles, toss, and serve hot.

NUTRIENTS, per serving:

Calories 338	Protein 8 gm	Carbohydrates 52 gm
Calcium 23 mg	Total fat 13 gm	Saturated fat 1.3 gm

EXCHANGES, not applicable

NOODLES WITH ALMONDS   *6 servings*

1 tablespoon non-dairy margarine
¼ cup slivered almonds
12 ounces broad noodles, cooked according to package directions

In a skillet, melt the margarine; saute the almonds for 1 minute then add to the cooked noodles; toss before serving.

NUTRIENTS, per serving:

Calories 281	Protein 9.5 gm	Carbohydrates 43 gm
Calcium 40 mg	Total fat 11 gm	Saturated fat 0.6 gm

EXCHANGES, per serving: 3 bread; 2 fat

NOODLE PUDDING   *8 servings*

1 tablespoon non-dairy margarine, softened
½ cup sugar
1 cup low-lactose cottage cheese
¼ cup raisins
rind of ½ lemon, grated
1 tablespoon lemon juice
2 eggs, separated
½ cup liquid egg substitute, added to the egg yolks
8 ounce broad noodles, cooked according to package directions

Blend the margarine with the sugar; add the cheese, raisins, lemon rind and lemon juice. Beat the egg yolks and egg substitute until thick, then add to the cheese mixture. Add the noodles. Beat the egg whites until stiff, then fold into cheese-egg mixture. Place in a greased 1½ quart casserole dish, set in a pan of hot water, and bake in a preheated 350° oven for 1 hour.

NUTRIENTS, per serving:

Calories 228	Protein 11 gm	Carbohydrates 37 gm
Calcium 38 mg	Total fat 4 gm	Saturated fat 1 gm

EXCHANGES, not applicable

VEGETABLE MANICOTTI   *8 servings*

Filling

10 ounces frozen chopped spinach, defrosted and drained
1 tablespoon vegetable oil
2 cups mashed tofu
1 egg
2 tablespoons egg substitute

Sauce

½ cup chopped onions
½ teaspoon minced garlic
1 tablespoon vegetable oil
4 cups canned tomatoes, drained and chopped
1 teaspoon oregano
16 manicotti shells

In a non-stick skillet, saute the spinach in the vegetable oil until limp. Combine the tofu egg and egg substitute. Add the chopped spinach to this mixture and set aside. To prepare the sauce, saute the chopped onions and garlic in the oil for 3 minutes. Add the drained tomatoes and oregano to the onions; simmer uncovered for 30 minutes. Stuff the manicotti shells with the spinach-tofu mixture. Pour one-half of the sauce into the bottom of a 9 x 13 inch baking dish; add the stuffed manicotti. Top with remaining sauce. Cover with foil, and bake in a preheated 350° oven for 35 minutes. Serve hot.

NUTRIENTS, per serving:

Calories 329	Protein 16 gm	Carbohydrates 50 gm
Calcium 163 mg	Total fat 8 gm	Saturated fat 1.4 gm

EXCHANGES, per serving: 1 meat; 3 bread; ½ fat

SPAGHETTI AND TUNA CASSEROLE   *8 servings*

¼ cup non-dairy margarine
2 tablespoons flour
pepper to taste
½ teaspoon minced garlic
1 cup lactose-reduced milk
13 ounces canned tuna (water pack, drained)
8 ounces spaghetti, cooked according to package directions, drained
1 cup non-dairy bread crumbs

Melt margarine in a saucepan; add flour, pepper, and garlic; blend well. Add the milk, stirring constantly until thickened. Add the tuna and the spaghetti. Place into a greased 1½ quart casserole dish and sprinkle with the bread crumbs. Bake in a 350° oven for 30 minutes, until brown.

NUTRIENTS, per serving:

Calories 332	Protein 19 gm	Carbohydrates 31 gm
Calcium 71 mg	Total fat 14 gm	Saturated fat 2.7 gm

EXCHANGES, per serving: 2 meat; 2 bread; 1 fat

MACARONI AND FRUIT SALAD   *6 servings*

2 cups unpeeled apples, cored and cubed
1 teaspoon lemon juice
1 cup seedless green grapes
1 cup chopped celery
8 ounces macaroni, cooked according to package directions and drained
¼ cup mayonnaise
¼ cup non-dairy or mock sour cream
½ cup coarsely chopped walnuts

Toss the apples with lemon juice; add the next 5 ingredients; mix gently; chill. Add the walnuts before serving.

NUTRIENTS, per serving:

Calories 310	Protein 10 gm	Carbohydrates 41 gm
Calcium 53 mg	Total fat 11 gm	Saturated fat 1 gm

EXCHANGES, per serving: 1 meat; 1 bread; 2 fruit; 1 fat

SOUPS

Soups offer convenient ways to serve important foods such as meat, fish, vegetables and pasta. And a number of creamy soups are presented which incorporate non-dairy products such as tofu and vegetable oils.

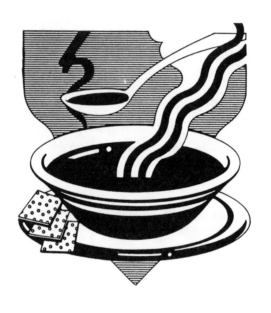

QUICK CREAM SOUPS   *6 servings*

<u>*Basic Sauce*</u>
2 tablespoons non-dairy margarine
6 tablespoons flour
6 cups soy milk
pepper to taste

Prepare the basic sauce by melting the margarine in a saucepan; stir in the flour and remove the pan from the heat. Add the milk all at once, heat, stirring slowly, to the boiling point (about 10 minutes). Add pepper. Use this base to prepare a variety of cream soups quickly:

<u>Cream of asparagus soup</u>: add ¾ pound cooked chopped asparagus; heat

<u>Cream of celery soup</u>: add 1 cup chopped celery and 1 tablespoon chopped sauteed onions; heat

<u>Cream of corn soup</u>: add 2 cans (1 pound each) creamed corn and 1 tablespoon chopped sauteed onions; heat

<u>Cream of pea soup</u>: add 2 cans (1 pound each) green peas; heat

<u>Cream of spinach soup</u>: add 10 ounces finely chopped fresh or frozen spinach; heat

<u>Cream of salmon soup</u>: add 6½ ounces canned salmon and 2 tablespoons chopped, minced and sauteed onions; heat and serve hot.

NUTRIENTS, per serving of basic sauce:

Calories 130	Protein 6.7 gm	Carbohydrates 7.8 gm
Calcium 6.3 mg	Total fat 7 gm	Saturated fat 2.6 gm

Addition of corn adds 70 calories and 16 gm carbohydrates to each serving; addition of peas adds 100 calories, 20 gm carbohydrates and 5 gm protein to each serving; addition of salmon adds 50 calories, 6 gm protein and 2 gm fat to each serving.

EXCHANGES, per serving of basic sauce: 1 meat; ½ bread; ½ fat

EXCHANGES, per serving of corn soup: 1 meat; 1½ bread; ½ fat

EXCHANGES, per serving of pea soup: 1 meat; 2 bread; ½ fat

EXCHANGES, per serving of salmon soup: 1½ meat; ½ bread

CREAM OF CARROT SOUP   *6 servings*

2 tablespoons non-dairy margarine
2½ cups diced carrots
½ cup chopped onions
2 cups diced, raw potatoes
4 cups chicken bouillon
½ teaspoon chopped dill weed
pepper to taste
¾ cup soy milk
¼ cup chopped parsley

Melt margarine in soup pot; add carrots and onions. Cover and saute over low heat for 5 minutes. Add potatoes, chicken bouillon, dill, and pepper; cover and simmer for 15 minutes until vegetables are tender. Puree soup in blender. Return to soup pot. Add soy milk and parsley; heat. Serve hot.

NUTRIENTS, per serving:

Calories 148   Protein 4 gm   Carbohydrates 23 gm
Calcium 41 mg   Total fat 5 gm   Saturated fat 1 gm

EXCHANGES, per serving: 1½ bread; 1 fat

ONION SOUP   *4 servings*

2 cups chopped onions
2 tablespoons vegetable oil
1 teaspoon minced garlic
5 cups water
½ cup white wine
pepper to taste
8 ounces tofu
2 tablespoons olive oil
2 teaspoons grated Parmesan cheese substitute

In a non-stick soup pot, saute the onions in the oil until soft and translucent; add the garlic and cook for 3 minutes. Add the water, white wine, and pepper; simmer about 40 minutes.

Slice the tofu into 1 inch cubes. Baste the tofu slices with the olive oil, then bake on an oiled baking sheet at 350° for 20 minutes, until crusty; add to the soup. Ladle soup into individual oven-proof bowls. Top with parmesan cheese substitute. Broil until the cheese melts, about 2 minutes. Serve hot.

NUTRIENTS, per serving:

Calories 200   Protein 7 gm   Carbohydrates 10 gm
Calcium 142 mg   Total fat 14 gm   Saturated fat 3 gm

EXCHANGES, per serving: ½ meat; 2 vegetable; 2 fat

TOMATO BISQUE   *4 servings*

2 medium onions, thinly sliced
½ teaspoon crushed garlic
2 tablespoons vegetable oil
2 cups cold water
1 tablespoon cornstarch
8 ounces tofu
2 pounds tomatoes, chopped
1 stalk celery, chopped
1 teaspoon parsley, chopped

In a non-stick soup pot, saute the onions and garlic in the oil until brown. Dissolve the cornstarch in 1 cup of cold water, and then pour into the sauteed onion and garlic mixture; stir to avoid lumps. Bring to boil over medium heat, stirring occasionally. Reduce heat, and simmer for 5 minutes.

Cut the tofu into small pieces. Puree the tomatoes in the blender, adding the tofu, piece by piece, until smooth. While the blender is still on, slowly add the onion-starch mixture. When the mixture is very smooth, return it to the sauce pan, add the chopped celery and the remaining cup of water. Heat gently for 5 minutes; serve hot with parsley garnish.

NUTRIENTS, per serving:

Calories 126	Protein 5 gm	Carbohydrates 10 gm
Calcium 85 mg	Total fat 8 gm	Saturated fat 1 gm

EXCHANGES, per serving: 2 vegetable; 1½ fat

CREAM OF TOMATO SOUP

4 servings

2 cups tomato juice
2 cups soy milk
1 tablespoon non-dairy margarine
1 tablespoon lemon juice
½ teaspoon dried basil
pepper to taste
¼ cup cornstarch
½ teaspoon parsley, chopped

Combine all ingredients except cornstarch in a saucepan. Stir until smooth while cooking over low heat. When margarine has melted, add cornstarch and cook 5 minutes more, with continual stirring. Serve hot, garnished with parsley.

NUTRIENTS, per serving:

Calories 130	Protein 5 gm	Carbohydrates 17 gm
Calcium 33 mg	Total fat 3.7 gm	Saturated fat 0.3 gm

EXCHANGES, per serving: 1 bread; ½ vegetable; 1 fat

FRESH VEGETABLE SOUP   *6 servings*

1 cup sliced carrots
1 cup sliced celery
1 cup diced potatoes
1 cup chopped onion
1 clove crushed garlic
1 cup fresh green beans, cut into 1 inch lengths
4 cups chopped fresh tomatoes
2 cups chicken bouillon
½ teaspoon dried basil
½ teaspoon dried thyme
pepper to taste
1 tablespoon chopped dill

Mix together all ingredients in a large soup pot. Bring to a boil, then cover and simmer 40 minutes. Add the dill just before serving. Serve hot.

NUTRIENTS, per serving:

| Calories 81 | Protein 3 gm | Carbohydrates 14 gm |
| Calcium 33 mg | Total fat 2.3 gm | Saturated fat 0.3 gm |

EXCHANGES, per serving: 1 bread; ½ fat

FRENCH ONION SOUP   *6 servings*

6 large, thinly sliced onions
1 tablespoon olive oil
6 cups beef bouillon
1/3 cup red or white wine
¼ cup grated hard cheese substitute, such as parmesan or cheddar
3 slices toasted non-dairy bread, halved

In a non-stick soup pot, brown onions in oil until limp. Cover and simmer slowly for 15 minutes. Pour in beef bouillon and simmer for 30 minutes. Ladle soup and wine into ovenproof casserole, cover and heat in a 350° oven for 30 minutes. Pour soup into individual bowls; add layer of bread and sprinkle with cheese. Serve hot.

NUTRIENTS, per serving:

Calories 160	Protein 8 gm	Carbohydrates 13 gm
Calcium 165 mg	Total fat 4.5 gm	Saturated fat 1.5 gm

EXCHANGES, per serving: ½ meat; ½ bread; 1 vegetable

CREAM OF ASPARAGUS SOUP   *4 servings*

4 cups chicken bouillon
2 cups chopped asparagus (fresh or frozen)
4 tablespoons chopped onion
1 cup non-pasteurized yogurt

Heat chicken bouillon; add asparagus and onion; cook until soft. Remove from heat and cool slightly; blend until smooth. Add yogurt; serve at once.

NUTRIENTS, per serving:

Calories 79	Protein 6 gm	Carbohydrates 10 gm
Calcium 132 mg	Total fat 2 gm	Saturated fat 1 gm

EXCHANGES, per serving: 2 vegetable; ½ fat

CUCUMBER/SPINACH SOUP   *6 servings*

3 cups chicken bouillon
2 cups chopped cucumbers (peeled and seeded)
1 chopped onion
1 clove minced garlic
1 cup chopped fresh spinach
1 cup non-pasteurized yogurt

Place chicken bouillon in saucepan. Add cucumbers, then add the onion and garlic. Bring to a boil, simmer about 30 minutes or until vegetables are soft. Add chopped spinach and cook 5 minutes more. Let cool slightly. In small batches, puree mixture in food processor or blender, adding the yogurt last. Serve well chilled.

NUTRIENTS, per serving:

Calories 48	Protein 3 gm	Carbohydrates 6 gm
Calcium 93 mg	Total fat 1 gm	Saturated fat 0.5 gm

EXCHANGES, per serving: 1 vegetable

CREAM OF BROCCOLI SOUP   *4 servings*

½ pound of fresh broccoli, cut into ½ inch pieces
2 tablespoons non-dairy margarine
¼ cup sifted flour
2 cups chicken bouillon
4 ounces fresh mushrooms, sliced
1 small potato, diced
½ cup soy milk
pepper to taste
1/8 teaspoon minced garlic

Steam the broccoli and do not drain; set aside. Melt margarine in pan over medium heat. Add flour, stirring to make a roux (2-4 minutes). Add the chicken bouillon, bring to a boil; lower heat, add the vegetables, soy milk and seasonings and heat until broccoli is tender, 10-15 minutes. Serve hot.

NUTRIENTS, per serving:

Calories 127	Protein 4 gm	Carbohydrates 13 gm
Calcium 37 mg	Total fat 7 gm	Saturated fat 3 gm

EXCHANGES, per serving: 1 bread; 1½ fat

CREAM OF ZUCCHINI SOUP   *4 servings*

2 cups chicken bouillon
3 cups sliced zucchini
2 chopped onions
1 clove minced garlic
¼ teaspoon curry powder
½ cup non-pasteurized yogurt (or ½ cup mock sour cream)
2 teaspoons lemon juice

Place bouillon, zucchini, onions, garlic and curry in a saucepan and bring to a boil. Reduce heat to low, cover and simmer until vegetables are tender. Cool slightly. Blend vegetables until smooth. Add yogurt (or sour cream) and lemon juice last. Serve well chilled.

NUTRIENTS, per serving:

Calories 79	Protein 6 gm	Carbohydrates 12 gm
Calcium 136 mg	Total fat 1.6 gm	Saturated fat 0.8 gm

EXCHANGES, per serving: 2 vegetable

POTATO BEAN SOUP   *6 servings*

1½ pounds potatoes, peeled and cut into 1 inch cubes
1 pound green beans cut into 1 inch lengths
6 cups water
3 tablespoons vegetable oil
2 teaspoons minced garlic
1 small chopped onion
pepper to taste
½ teaspoon chopped parsley

Cook the potatoes in the water (in a covered pot) for about 15 minutes; add the green beans and cook (uncovered) for another 15 minutes. In a separate skillet, saute the garlic and onion in the oil for about 5 minutes, then add this mixture to the potato bean soup. Season. Serve hot, garnished with parsley.

NUTRIENTS, per serving:

Calories 133	Protein 1.8 gm	Carbohydrates 12 gm
Calcium 33 mg	Total fat 9 gm	Saturated fat 1 gm

EXCHANGES, per serving: 1 bread; 2 fat

POTATO LEEK SOUP   *4 servings*

4 medium potatoes, peeled and diced
2 large leeks, sliced thin
2 stalks celery, diced
1 teaspoon crushed garlic
3 cups water
pepper to taste
2 tablespoons non-dairy margarine
2 tablespoons cornstarch
1 cup chicken bouillon

Place potatoes, leeks, celery, dill weed, water and pepper in a pot. Simmer until potatoes are tender, about 20 minutes. In a separate pan, melt margarine and stir in flour. Cook until thickened, while stirring. Gradually add chicken bouillon and stir until smooth, then add this mixture to the potato soup, mixing well. Cook for several minutes; serve hot.

<u>NUTRIENTS</u>, per serving:

Calories 123	Protein 2 gm	Carbohydrates 12 gm
Calcium 20 mg	Total fat 8 gm	Saturated fat 1.7 gm

<u>EXCHANGES</u>, per serving: 1 bread; 2 fat

VICHYSSOISE   *6 servings*

1 medium onion, minced
1 teaspoon non-dairy margarine
3 cups chicken bouillon
3 medium potatoes (peeled and diced)
white pepper to taste
1 teaspoon chopped scallions

In a non-stick skillet, brown onions in margarine and set aside. Add the bouillon and potatoes to the onions; add pepper and bring to a boil; cover and simmer for 25 minutes. Cool. Beat in a blender until thoroughly combined. Chill; serve garnished with chopped scallions.

<u>NUTRIENTS</u>, per serving:

Calories 60	Protein 2 gm	Carbohydrates 8 gm
Calcium 22 mg	Total fat 2.7 gm	Saturated fat 0.6 gm

<u>EXCHANGES</u>, per serving: ½ bread; ½ fat

CLAM CHOWDER   *6 servings*

2 cups raw potatoes, peeled and diced
2 cups chicken bouillon
½ cup clam juice
2 cups canned clams, minced

Add diced potatoes to bouillon and bring to a boil; cover and simmer
for 25 minutes. Liquify in a blender. Add the claim juice and clams;
heat just to boiling and serve hot.

NUTRIENTS, per serving:

Calories 165	Protein 16 gm	Carbohydrates 15 gm
Calcium 76 mg	Total fat 4.5 gm	Saturated fat 1 gm

EXCHANGES, per serving: 2 meat; 1 bread

FISH CHOWDER   *6 servings*

1 chopped onion
1 chopped green pepper
1 clove minced garlic
1 teaspoon vegetable oil
4 cups stewed tomatoes
½ teaspoon dried thyme
2 cups dry white wine
2 cups water
2 tablespoons lemon juice
2 potatoes, peeled and diced
2 pounds fish (red snapper, blue fish or haddock)

Spray saute pan with non-stick cooking spray. Brown onion, green pepper and garlic in oil. Add tomatoes, thyme, wine, water and lemon juice. Bring to a boil, simmer 30 minutes. Add potatoes, cook 15 minutes. Cut fish in 1 inch cubes, add to sauce and cook 2-3 minutes or just until fish flakes.

<u>NUTRIENTS</u>, per serving:

Calories 278	Protein 40 gm	Carbohydrates 13 gm
Calcium 111 mg	Total fat 4 gm	Saturated fat 0.8 gm

<u>EXCHANGES</u>, per serving: 5 meat; 1 bread

BORSCHT   *4 servings*

½ cup chopped onion
1 pound canned, sliced beets, plus juice
2 cups shredded cabbage
½ cup chopped carrot
½ cup diced potato
2 tablespoons vinegar
4 cups beef bouillon
¼ cup non-dairy sour cream or non-pasteurized yogurt

Combine all ingredients except sour cream (or yogurt) and simmer for 1 hour, until vegetables are tender. Cool slightly, then blend small amounts in blender. Return blended mixture to pot and heat. Serve with 1 tablespoon sour cream (or yogurt) in center of each serving.

<u>NUTRIENTS</u>, per serving:

Calories 196	Protein 8 gm	Carbohydrates 38 gm
Calcium 140 mg	Total fat 2.5 gm	Saturated fat 0.8 gm

<u>EXCHANGES</u>, per serving: 2 bread; 1 vegetable; ½ fat

BEAN AND PASTA SOUP   *6 servings*

2 tablespoons olive oil
¾ cup chopped green peppers
¾ cup chopped onion
½ teaspoon crushed garlic
¼ cup chopped celery
¾ cup finely sliced carrots
4 medium tomatoes, peeled and chopped
½ teaspoon dried oregano
pepper to taste
4 cups beef bouillon
3 cups water
2 cups macaroni, cooked according to package instructions and drained
1 10 ounce can of kidney beans

Add the oil to a large pot; add the next five vegetables and cook for 10-12 minutes at moderate heat. Add the tomatoes, oregano, pepper, beef bouillon and water; continue to simmer for 15 minutes. Add the cooked macaroni and the kidney beans. Heat for an additional 10 minutes. Serve hot.

NUTRIENTS, per serving:

Calories 246	Protein 8.7 gm	Carbohydrates 40 gm
Calcium 31.5 mg	Total fat 6 gm	Saturated fat 1.0 gm

EXCHANGES, per serving: 2 bread; 2 vegetable; 1 fat

CHILLED FRUIT SOUP

4 servings

1 pound canned pitted dark cherries, including liquid (or 1½ cups frozen raspberries)
2 teaspoons lemon juice
¼ teaspoon cinnamon
2 tablespoons sugar
5 ounces tofu, drained
½ cup grape juice
¼ cup red wine
4 thin lemon slices

Combine the first four ingredients in a saucepan; simmer for 5 minutes. Cool; puree the mixture, then filter through coarse cheese cloth; set aside. In a blender, whip the tofu with the cherry puree, the grape juice and the wine. Serve well chilled, garnished with thin lemon slices.

NUTRIENTS, per serving:

Calories 113	Protein 2.5 gm	Carbohydrates 23 gm
Calcium 42 mg	Total fat 1.2 gm	Saturated fat 0.3 gm

EXCHANGES, per serving: not applicable

APRICOT SOUP   *6 servings*

2 cups dried apricots
3 cups water
2 tablespoons sugar
¼ teaspoon cinnamon
1 teaspoon lemon juice
¾ cup non-dairy cream
1½ cups water

Simmer apricots in the 3 cups water, in a covered pot, for 30 minutes; puree this mixture in a blender. Add the remaining ingredients. Heat (do not boil) if served hot; chill if served cold. Garnish with thin lemon slices.

NUTRIENTS, per serving:

Calories 81	Protein 0.4 gm	Carbohydrates 15 gm
Calcium 5.4 mg	Total fat 4 gm	Saturated fat 0.0 gm

EXCHANGES, not applicable

FISH

Fish and shellfish are excellent sources of protein and the B-vitamins. And the judicious use of non-dairy cream and soy milk permit those sensitive to lactose to enjoy such dishes as creamed fish and fish Newburg. The recipes using canned fish employ water-pack varieties; if oil-pack is used, first rinse the fish with water.

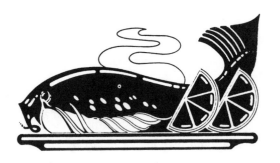

FISH VERONIQUE   *6 servings*

2 pounds fish fillets (flounder or haddock)
pepper to taste
¼ cup dry white wine
1 cup water
2 tablespoons finely chopped onion
1 tablespoon lemon juice
1 cup seedless green or white grapes
6 tablespoons white sauce (see section on sauces and gravies)

Sprinkle fish with pepper, place fish in 10 inch skillet; add wine, water, onions and lemon juice. Heat to boiling, cover and simmer until fish flakes easily with fork (4 to 5 minutes). Remove with slotted spoon to heatproof platter; keep warm. Add grapes to liquid in skillet. Heat to boiling; simmer uncovered 3 minutes; remove grapes. Boil remaining liquid until reduced to 1 cup; save. Drain excess liquid from fish; spoon 6 tablespoons white cream-style sauce over fish. Broil fish until the sauce thickens; serve with grape garnish.

NUTRIENTS, per tablespoon:

Calories 187	Protein 34.5 gm	Carbohydrates 2.9 gm
Calcium 62.5 mg	Total fat 2.3 gm	Saturated fat 0.3 gm

EXCHANGES, per tablespoon: 5 meat

FISH WITH SOUR CREAM (OR YOGURT)   *4 servings*

1 pound fish fillets (haddock or flounder)
4 ounce mushrooms, sliced
1 small onion, chopped
1 tablespoon non-dairy margarine
pepper to taste
½ cup non-dairy sour cream (non-pasteurized yogurt may be substituted)
2 tablespoons dry dairy-free bread crumbs
paprika

Cut into serving pieces; pat dry. Arrange in ungreased oblong baking dish. Saute the mushrooms and onion in non-dairy margarine in a non-stick skillet for about 3 minutes. Spoon mushroom mixture over fish; sprinkle with pepper. Spread sour cream substitute (or yogurt) over mushroom mixture. Sprinkle with bread crumbs. Cook uncovered in 350° oven until fish flakes easily with fork, 25 to 30 minutes. Garnish with paprika.

<u>NUTRIENTS</u>, per tablespoon:

Calories 233	Protein 27.5 gm	Carbohydrates 5.8 gm
Calcium 62.8 mg	Total fat 11 gm	Saturated fat 4.4 gm

<u>EXCHANGES</u>, per tablespoon: 4 meat; 1 vegetable;

STUFFED SOLE *6 servings*

½ pound mushrooms, sliced
2 teaspoons vegetable oil
½ pound fresh spinach, chopped
¼ teaspoon garlic powder
¼ teaspoon dried oregano
1½ pounds sole fillets (6 pieces)
4 teaspoons lemon juice
2 tablespoons grated mozzarella cheese substitute
paprika

Brown mushrooms in oil until limp. Add spinach, and cook for one minute; remove from heat and drain. Add garlic powder and oregano. Place one quarter of the mixture in the center of each fillet; roll and place in a baking dish sprayed with non-stick cooking spray. Sprinkle with lemon juice and bake in a 425° oven for 15 minutes; sprinkle with cheese and bake an additional 5 minutes. Garnish with paprika.

NUTRIENTS, per serving:

Calories 150	Protein 28 gm	Carbohydrates 0.5 gm
Calcium 63 mg	Total fat 3 gm	Saturated fat 1.0 gm

EXCHANGES, per serving: 4 meat

BAKED FISH   *4 servings*

½ cup onion, chopped
2 tablespoons margarine, melted
1 pound perch fillets
1 tablespoon lemon juice
¼ teaspoon paprika
2 tablespoons non-dairy bread crumbs
1 tablespoon chopped parsley

Saute chopped onion in 1 tablespoon margarine until transparent. Lightly grease a shallow baking pan. Place fillets in a single layer, skin side down in pan. Mix remaining margarine, sauteed onion, lemon juice and paprika. Spoon over fillets. Bake at 350° until fish flakes easily, about 20 minutes. Garnish each serving with bread crumbs and parsley.

NUTRIENTS, per serving:

Calories 194	Protein 26 gm	Carbohydrates 3 gm
Calcium 154 mg	Total fat 8 gm	Saturated fat 0.9 gm

EXCHANGES, per serving: 4 meat

CURRIED FISH

4 servings

1 medium-sized onion, chopped
½ teaspoon minced garlic
1 tablespoon non-dairy margarine
1 teaspoon curry powder
2 medium-sized tomatoes, sliced
1 tablespoon lemon juice
1 pound fish fillets (halibut, flounder or blue fish), cut into serving size
  pieces
1 tablespoon chopped parsley

Saute the onion and garlic for 3-5 minutes in the margarine in a non-stick skillet. Add the curry powder; mix well. Add tomatoes and saute gently until tender; crush the tomatoes, then add the lemon juice. Cook on medium heat for 4 to 5 minutes, then add the fish, covering the fish with the sauce. When the sauce starts to boil, cover and simmer for 10 minutes. Serve sprinkled with parsley.

NUTRIENTS, per serving:

Calories 170	Protein 26.5 gm	Carbohydrates 4.8 gm
Calcium 31 mg	Total fat 4.7 gm	Saturated fat 0.9 gm

EXCHANGES, per serving: 3½ meat; 1 vegetable

CREAMED FISH   *4 servings*

4 ounces mushrooms, sliced
1 medium onion, finely chopped
2 tablespoons non-dairy margarine
1 pound fish fillet (flounder, pollack or haddock)
½ cup dry white wine
1 tablespoon lemon juice
1 tablespoon flour
¼ cup non-dairy cream
¼ teaspoon white pepper

Cook and stir mushrooms and onions in 1 tablespoons margarine in non-stick skillet until mushrooms are tender, about 3 minutes; remove from skillet. Place fish in skillet; add wine, lemon juice and just enough water to cover fish. Heat to boiling; reduce heat, cover, and simmer until fish flakes easily with fork, 4 to 5 minutes. Remove fish with slotted spoon to platter; keep warm. Heat liquid in skillet to boiling; boil until reduced to 1 cup (about 15 minutes). Pour liquid into measuring cup; reserve. Heat 1 tablespoon margarine in skillet until melted; stir in flour. Cook and stir 1 minute; remove from heat. Stir in reserved liquid and the cream. Heat to boiling, stirring constantly. Stir in mushrooms, onions, and pepper. Pour sauce over fish; serve hot.

NUTRIENTS, per serving:

Calories 228	Protein 29 gm	Carbohydrates 5.6 gm
Calcium 57 mg	Total fat 9 gm	Saturated fat 1.5 gm

EXCHANGES, not applicable

FISH FLORENTINE
6 servings

2 tablespoons non-dairy margarine
2 tablespoons flour
Dash of ground nutmeg
white pepper to season
1 cup soy milk
10 ounces frozen chopped spinach, thawed and drained
1 tablespoon lemon juice
1 pound fish fillets (haddock, halibut or flounder)
2 tablespoons grated non-dairy parmesan cheese (optional)
1/8 teaspoon paprika

Melt margarine over low heat; blend in flour, nutmeg and pepper. Cook over low heat stirring constantly, until mixture is smooth and bubbly; remove from heat. Stir in soy milk. Heat to boiling; reduce heat to simmer and stir until thickened, about 3 minutes.

Place spinach in a greased baking dish, sprinkle with lemon juice. Arrange fish on spinach. Spread sauce over fish and spinach. Cook uncovered in 350° oven until fish flakes easily with fork, 20 to 25 minutes. Sprinkle with cheese substitute and paprika before serving.

NUTRIENTS, per serving:

Calories 193	Protein 25 gm	Carbohydrates 5.5 gm
Calcium 235 mg	Total fat 8 gm	Saturated fat 2 gm

EXCHANGES, per serving: 3 meat; 1 vegetable

SAUTEED FISH IN PUNGENT SAUCE   *8 servings*

¼ cup vegetable oil
1½ pounds fish fillets (haddock, for example)cut into serving pieces
¾ cup water
2 carrots, thinly sliced
2 small onions, sliced
1 small green pepper cut into rings
1 clove garlic, minced
1 tablespoon packed brown sugar
¾ teaspoon ground ginger
1/3 cup vinegar
2 tablespoons cornstarch

Heat oil in skillet until hot. Pat fish dry and cook over medium heat until fish flakes easily with fork (about 10 minutes). Heat water, carrots, onions, green pepper, garlic, brown sugar and ginger to boiling; reduce heat. Cover and simmer 5 minutes. Mix vinegar and cornstarch together and stir into vegetables. Heat to boiling, stirring constantly, for 1 minute then pour over fish. Serve with rice.

NUTRIENTS, per serving:

| Calories 170 | Protein 20.7 gm | Carbohydrates 3.6 gm |
| Calcium 40 mg | Total fat 7.6 gm | Saturated fat 1 gm |

EXCHANGES, per serving: 3 meat; ½ vegetable

FISH SALAD   *4 servings*

1 pound flounder, cooked and flaked
2 tablespoons lemon juice
½ cup chopped celery
pepper to taste
¼ teaspoon dried dillweed
½ cup mayonnaise

Mix flaked fish, lemon juice, celery and spices; add mayonnaise and mix thoroughly. Serve on bed of lettuce.

NUTRIENTS, per serving:

Calories 223	Protein 26 gm	Carbohydrates 2 gm
Calcium 25 mg	Total fat 11.6 gm	Saturated fat 2.4 gm

EXCHANGES, per serving: 3½ meat

TUNA ALASKA   *2 servings*

7 ounces canned tuna
2 tablespoons non-pasteurized yogurt
1 tablespoon mayonnaise
¼ teaspoon dried dill weed
2 tablespoons lemon juice
1 tablespoon minced green onion
pepper to taste
2 slices non-dairy bread
1 egg white

Preheat broiler. Make a tuna salad with first seven ingredients. Toast 2 slices of bread. Spread tuna on toast and cover completely with beaten egg white. Broil the sandwich until the meringue is cooked and brown.

NUTRIENTS, per serving:

Calories 260	Protein 28 gm	Carbohydrates 15 mg
Calcium 71 mg	Total fat 8.8 gm	Saturated fat 1.8 gm

EXCHANGES, per serving: 3½ meat; 1 bread

SALMON NEWBURG   *4 servings*

2 tablespoons non-dairy margarine
1 tablespoon grated onion
3 tablespoons flour
pepper to taste
1 teaspoon paprika
1½ cups soy milk
1/8 teaspoon tabasco sauce
1 pound salmon, drained and flaked
1 tablespoon chopped parsley
½ cup egg substitute
¼ cup non-dairy cream
3 tablespoons cognac

Melt margarine in sauce pan; add onion and saute for 5 minutes.
Blend in flour, pepper and paprika. Gradually stir in soy milk and
tabasco sauce. Cook over low heat, stirring until thick and smooth.
Stir in salmon and parsley and simmer for 3 minutes. Blend egg
substitute with cream and cognac; add to salmon mixture, and cook
for 2 minutes longer. Serve with rice or noodles.

NUTRIENTS, per serving:

Calories 401	Protein 33 gm	Carbohydrates 12 gm
Calcium 356 mg	Total fat 16 gm	Saturated fat 2.6 gm

EXCHANGES, per serving: 4½ meat; 1 bread

SALMON LOAF   *6 servings*

1 pound canned salmon, with bones mashed
½ cup dairy-free breadcrumbs
¼ cup chopped scallions
2 tablespoons chopped fresh parsley
½ teaspoon celery salt
pepper to taste
1 egg, well beaten
½ teaspoon non-dairy margarine
1 cup canned tomato sauce

Drain and flake salmon. Add crumbs, scallions, parsley, celery salt, pepper and egg; mix well and place into a greased 5 x 9 inch loaf pan. Bake at 350° for 30 minutes. Serve with heated tomato sauce.

NUTRIENTS, per serving:

Calories 189	Protein 17.6 gm	Carbohydrates 10 gm
Calcium 210 mg	Total fat 8.5 gm	Saturated fat 1.7 gm

EXCHANGES, per serving: 2 meat; ½ bread

CREAMED SALMON   *6 servings*

1 pound canned salmon, with bones mashed
2 cups white sauce (pg. 67)
¼ teaspoon chopped parsley

Blend the ingredients in a saucepan; heat just to boiling and serve over rice, garnished with parsley.

NUTRIENTS, per serving:

Calories 217	Protein 24 gm	Carbohydrates 4.4 gm
Calcium 280 mg	Total fat 14 gm	Saturated fat 2.8 gm

EXCHANGES, per serving: 3 meat

SALMON-CUCUMBER SALAD   *4 servings*

2 cucumbers
pepper to taste
1 pound canned salmon, drained and flaked
¾ cup non-dairy or mock sour cream
1 tablespoon lemon juice
2 tablespoons minced green onions

Quarter cucumbers, seed, and cut in thin slices. Sprinkle with pepper. Drain well and mix lightly with salmon. Mix mock sour cream with lemon juice. Pour over salmon mixture and garnish with onion.

NUTRIENTS, per serving:

Calories 320	Protein 30 gm	Carbohydrates 2.1 gm
Calcium 277 mg	Total fat 8 gm	Saturated fat 1.8 gm

EXCHANGES, per serving: 4 meat

SALMON DIVAN

4 servings

20 ounces frozen broccoli spears
2 tablespoons non-dairy margarine
2 tablespoons flour
pepper to taste
1 cup soy milk
1 tablespoon sherry
1 pound canned salmon, drained and flaked

Cook broccoli as directed on package; drain and put in shallow baking dish. Melt margarine and blend in flour and pepper. Gradually add milk and cook, stirring, until thickened. Add sherry. Spread salmon on broccoli and pour sauce over top; bake in 450° oven 15 to 20 minutes.

NUTRIENTS, per serving:

Calories 268	Protein 27 gm	Carbohydrates 8.5 gm
Calcium 315 mg	Total fat 15 gm	Saturated fat 2.8 gm

EXCHANGES, per serving: 3½ meat; 1½ vegetable

SALMON PUFFS

3 servings

1 can (6½ ounces) salmon
½ cup mayonnaise
½ teaspoon lemon juice
2 egg whites, stiffly beaten
3 slices non-dairy bread, toasted
3 lemon wedges

Blend together the salmon, mayonnaise and lemon juice; fold in the egg whites. Place a third of the mixture on each slice of toast, place under a broiler for 20-30 seconds until browned. Serve hot with lemon wedges.

NUTRIENTS, per serving:

Calories 296	Protein 16 gm	Carbohydrates 15 gm
Calcium 176 mg	Total fat 18 gm	Saturated fat 3.9 gm

EXCHANGES, per serving: 2 meat; 1 bread; 1½ fat

SHRIMP PUFFS   *3 dozen puffs*

2 egg whites
½ cup grated cheddar cheese substitute
¼ teaspoon paprika
1 cup mayonnaise
20 medium shrimp

Preheat broiler, whip egg whites until stiff. Fold in cheese, paprika, mayonnaise, chopped shrimp; heap lightly on crackers. Broil until lightly browned.

NUTRIENTS, per 3 puffs:

Calories 120	Protein 7.5 gm	Carbohydrates 1.8 gm
Calcium 81 mg	Total fat 8.7 gm	Saturated fat 2.4 gm

EXCHANGES, per serving: 1 meat; 1 fat

DILLED SHRIMP SALAD   *3 servings*

1 cup cooked shrimp, chopped
½ cup chopped celery
2 tablespoons chopped green onion
1 teaspoon dried dill weed
2 tablespoons green peppers, finely chopped
1 tablespoon lemon juice
2 tablespoons non-dairy cream
2 tablespoons mayonnaise
pepper to taste

Blend all ingredients in a food processor until smooth. Serve well chilled with crackers or pita bread.

NUTRIENTS, per serving:

Calories 175	Protein 20 gm	Carbohydrates 2 gm
Calcium 61 mg	Total fat 8.8 gm	Saturated fat 1.3 gm

EXCHANGES, not applicable

CHILLED SHRIMP WITH PEA PODS   *6 servings*

4 cups water
8 ounces fresh or frozen raw shrimp, peeled and deveined
6 ounces frozen Chinese pea pods
8 ounces tofu, cut into 1 inch slices
1 green onion, finely chopped
2 tablespoons soy sauce
1 tablespoon sesame oil

Heat water to boiling. Add shrimp and simmer until shrimp is pink, about 5 minutes; drain. Cook pea pods as directed on package; drain. Place tofu, shrimp, pea pods and green onion in bowl. Add soy sauce and sesame oil; mix gently. Serve with rice.

NUTRIENTS, per serving:

Calories 92	Protein 16 gm	Carbohydrates 4 gm
Calcium 106 mg	Total fat 4.3 gm	Saturated fat 0.8 gm

EXCHANGES, per serving: 2 meat

SCALLOPS SUPREME   *4 servings*

¼ cup minced onion
1 cup sliced mushrooms
2 tablespoons finely chopped green onion
1 clove minced garlic
1 teaspoon vegetable oil
1 pound scallops
½ cup flour
½ cup dry white wine
¼ cup water
1/8 teaspoon dried dill weed
pepper to taste
2 teaspoons lemon juice
¼ cup non dairy cream

Cook onions, mushrooms, garlic and oil, in a pan coated with non-stick cooking spray, for 5 minutes. Cut scallops into ½ inch pieces, dip in flour and add to pan to brown lightly. Add wine, water and dill and simmer 5 minutes. Remove vegetables and scallops from this sauce and place into four individual serving dishes. Cook sauce until thick, add pepper, lemon juice and cream. Pour sauce over each serving; heat in a 350° oven for 15 minutes. Serve hot.

NUTRIENTS, per serving:

Calories 169	Protein 18 gm	Carbohydrates 8.4 gm
Calcium 26 mg	Total fat 4 gm	Saturated fat 0.3 gm

EXCHANGES, not applicable

POULTRY

Poultry is an excellent source of protein and the B-vitamins. While the recipes presented here are with chicken, variations based on turkey offer numerous possibilities for interesting changes. The recipes given use skinned chicken parts to further reduce the fat content of the dish.

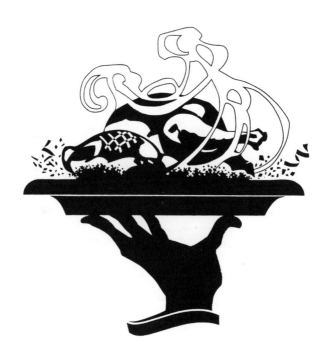

CHICKEN IN YOGURT SAUCE

6 servings

3 pounds chicken, cut into eighths
2 tablespoons flour
3 tablespoons vegetable oil
½ cup non-pasteurized yogurt
¼ cup chicken bouillon

Dust the chicken pieces with flour; heat oil in a skillet coated with non-sticking cooking spray and saute the chicken for about 20 minutes. Drain the fat and let cool for 10 minutes, then add the yogurt and chicken bouillon. Simmer for a few minutes. Serve over rice.

NUTRIENTS, per serving:

Calories 171	Protein 19 gm	Carbohydrates 3 gm
Calcium 42 mg	Total fat 9 gm	Saturated fat 1.8 gm

EXCHANGES, per serving: 2½ meat

CHICKEN IN COGNAC

4 servings

4 chicken breasts, boned
2 teaspoons margarine
1 cup sliced mushrooms
½ teaspoon garlic
½ cup cognac
½ cup chicken bouillon
1 teaspoon cornstarch
¼ cup non-dairy cream
2 teaspoons lemon juice

Brown chicken breasts slowly on both sides in a pan coated with non-sticking cooking spray.   Remove from pan, add margarine, mushrooms and garlic and stir until lightly browned. Return chicken to pan, add cognac. Simmer for 10 minutes or until chicken breasts are done (when pierced with fork, juices should not be pink). Stir together chicken bouillon and cornstarch, add to pan juices and mix well. Boil 1-2 minutes until thick, stir in cream and heat briefly until sauce thickens slightly; add lemon juice and serve.

NUTRIENTS, per serving:

Calories 296	Protein 27 gm	Carbohydrates 19 gm
Calcium 26.5 mg	Total fat 6.3 gm	Saturated fat 1.7 gm

EXCHANGES, not applicable

CHICKEN CORDON BLEU   *4 servings*

4 half chicken breasts, skinned and boned
4 thin slices turkey ham, about 1 x 3 inches
4 thin slices non-dairy mozzarella cheese (about 2 ounces total weight)
2 teaspoons oil
¼ teaspoon dried thyme
2/3 cup chicken bouillon
¼ cup cognac
¼ cup lemon juice
pepper to taste

Pound chicken breasts until approximately ¼ inch thick. On top of each flat breast, place a slice of ham and a slice of cheese. Roll up chicken, tuck in ends and secure with toothpicks. Heat oil in non-stick pan and brown chicken rolls on all sides. Sprinkle with thyme and pour bouillon over rolls. Cover and simmer 15 minutes. Remove chicken breasts and keep warm. Increase heat, add wine, lemon juice and pepper sauce to half its original volume. Pour over chicken breasts. Serve with rice.

<u>NUTRIENTS</u>, per serving:

Calories 358	Protein 37.5 gm	Carbohydrates 13 gm
Calcium 119 mg	Total fat 8.8 gm	Saturated fat 3 gm

<u>EXCHANGES</u>, per serving: 5 meat; 1 bread

CHICKEN TORTILLAS   *4 servings*

8 tortillas
2 teaspoons vegetable oil
½ cup chopped onions
½ cup chopped green pepper
1 cup cooked chicken, diced
1 teaspoon chili powder
2 teaspoons Worcestershire sauce
1 cup non-pasteurized yogurt (or non-dairy sour cream)
1 cup chopped tomato

Wrap the tortillas in foil and heat at 350° for 5 minutes. Saute the onions and peppers in the oil until the onions are soft. Add the chicken, chili and Worcestershire sauce and heat for 2-3 minutes. Fill the tortillas with the chicken mixture, spread with two tablespoons each of the yogurt and tomato. Two tortillas make a serving.

<u>NUTRIENTS</u>, per serving:

Calories 243	Protein 15 gm	Carbohydrates 27 gm
Calcium 153 mg	Total fat 8 gm	Saturated fat 2 gm

<u>EXCHANGES</u>, per serving: 1½ meat; 2 bread

CHICKEN IN CREAM SAUCE   *6 servings*

3 pounds chicken, cut into eighths
3 tablespoons vegetable oil
1 cup non-dairy cream
¼ cup cognac

Brown the chicken pieces in a large skillet; drain oil. Add the cream and cognac and cook for 45 minutes. Serve with peas or asparagus.

NUTRIENTS, per serving:

Calories 231	Protein 17 gm	Carbohydrates 10 gm
Calcium 9 mg	Total fat 14 gm	Saturated fat 1.3 gm

EXCHANGES, not applicable

CHICKEN FRICASSEE   *4 servings*

3 pounds chicken parts
¾ cup flour
½ teaspoon paprika
pepper to taste
3 tablespoons vegetable oil
½ cup brown sauce (pg. 75) diluted with 2 tablespoons water

Coat the chicken with the mixture of flour and seasonings. Heat oil in non-stick skillet and brown the chicken. Remove to baking dish, cover with sauce and bake in a 350° preheated oven for 50 minutes. Serve with asparagus spears.

NUTRIENTS, per serving:

Calories 283	Protein 26 gm	Carbohydrates 16 gm
Calcium 21 mg	Total fat 18 gm	Saturated fat 4 gm

EXCHANGES, per serving: 3 meat; 1 bread; ½ fat

CHICKEN PAPRIKASH I

4 servings

1 three pound chicken, cut into eighths
1 cup chicken bouillon
1 onion, chopped
2 small potatoes, cubed
1 carrot sliced
2 tablespoons paprika
3 tablespoons flour
1 cup tomato sauce
1 cup non-dairy cream
½ teaspoon chopped parsley

In a skillet coated with non-stick spray, saute the chicken until brown on each side; save for later. Add the bouillon, onion, potatoes and carrot to the skillet and cook over low heat for 10 minutes, stirring occasionally. Add the paprika; remove from heat and stir in the flour and tomato sauce; simmer for 15 minutes. Add the chicken pieces and cook for 30 minutes. Just before serving, blend in the cream substitute. Garnish with parsley. Serve with cooked noodles.

NUTRIENTS, per serving:

Calories 193	Protein 25 gm	Carbohydrates 9 gm
Calcium 33 mg	Total fat 7 gm	Saturated fat 0.5 gm

EXCHANGES, not applicable

CHICKEN PAPRIKASH II   *6 servings*

4 pounds chicken parts
2 tablespoons paprika
2 tablespoons salad oil
1 onion, sliced thin
1 cup chicken bouillon
1 tablespoon cornstarch
¼ cup water

Wash and dry the chicken parts. Sprinkle heavily with paprika. Heat oil in a non-stick pan; saute the onion until transparent. Add chicken and brown lightly, turning constantly. Add bouillon. Cover and simmer for 1 hour or until chicken parts are tender. Stir cornstarch into water, add several tablespoons of the sauce from the chicken; continue to stir and cook until gravy is thickened. Serve with cooked noodles.

NUTRIENTS, per serving:

Calories 144	Protein 18 gm	Carbohydrates 3 gm
Calcium 17 mg	Total fat 6 gm	Saturated fat 1 gm

EXCHANGES, per serving: 2½ meat

OVEN-FRIED CHICKEN   *4 servings*

3 pounds chicken parts
½ cup salad oil
pepper to taste
1 cup finely crushed bran flakes

Dip each chicken piece in oil; drain and sprinkle each piece with pepper and roll in crushed crumbs. Arrange in greased, shallow baking dish, leaving space between pieces; cover tightly with foil. Bake in 400° oven for 45 minutes or until chicken is tender; uncover for last 15 minutes to brown. Serve with rice.

NUTRIENTS, per serving:

Calories 268	Protein 27 gm	Carbohydrates 6 gm
Calcium 13 mg	Total fat 26.6 gm	Saturated fat 2 gm

EXCHANGES, per serving: 4 meat; 1 fat

CHICKEN A LA KING   *6 servings*

¾ cup non-dairy margarine
3 tablespoons flour
1½ cup chicken bouillon
½ cup dry white wine
1 teaspoon chopped garlic
pepper to taste
2½ cups cooked, diced chicken
2 tablespoons vegetable oil
½ cup chopped green pepper
½ cup chopped red pepper
1 cup sliced mushrooms

Melt the margarine, add flour (stirring constantly) then add the chicken bouillon, wine, garlic and pepper; heat while stirring until smooth and thickened. Add the sauce to the chicken. In a separate non-stick pan, saute the peppers and mushrooms in the oil; add to the chicken mixture and mix gently. Serve hot over rice.

NUTRIENTS, per serving:

| Calories 245 | Protein 17 gm | Carbohydrates 5.8 gm |
| Calcium 18 mg | Total fat 20 gm | Saturated fat 3.5 gm |

EXCHANGES, per serving: 1 meat; 2 fat; 1 vegetable

CHICKEN AND RICE CASSEROLE   *8 servings*

4 tablespoons non-dairy margarine
6 pounds chicken, cut into eighths
1 cup uncooked rice
1 cup non-dairy cream
1 cup chicken bouillon
pepper to taste

In a skillet, melt the margarine and saute the chicken pieces until brown on both sides; remove the chicken. Add the rice, cream substitute and bouillon; cover and bake in preheated 375° oven for 20 minutes. Serve with a green vegetable.

NUTRIENTS, per serving:

| Calories 172 | Protein 25 gm | Carbohydrates 12 gm |
| Calcium 1.5 mg | Total fat 10 gm | Saturated fat 0.4 gm |

EXCHANGES, not applicable

CHICKEN CROQUETTES   *6 servings*

2 tablespoons non-dairy margarine
½ cup flour
1 cup lactose-reduced milk
2 cups cooked chicken, chopped
¼ cup egg substitute plus 1 tablespoon
pepper to taste
1 cup non-dairy breadcrumbs
2 tablespoons vegetable oil

In a skillet, melt the margarine and blend in ¼ cup of the flour. Add the milk and cook at low heat for 2-3 minutes (do not boil). Set aside to cool. When at room temperature, add the chicken and ¼ cup egg substitute and pepper. Form into 4-inch patties, brush with the remaining egg substitute, roll in the breadcrumbs and saute in hot oil until golden brown. Serve with a green vegetable.

NUTRIENTS, per serving::

Calories 274	Protein 18 gm	Carbohydrates 20 gm
Calcium 81 mg	Total fat 13 gm	Saturated fat 2.7 gm

EXCHANGES, per serving: 2 meat; 1 bread; ½ fat

CHICKEN TETRAZZINI   *6 servings*

3 tablespoons non-dairy margarine
4 tablespoons flour
1¾ cups chicken bouillon
2 tablespoons egg substitute
¾ cup soy milk
4 tablespoons dry sherry
1 cup mushrooms, sliced
3 cups chicken, shredded
8 ounce package of spaghetti (cooked according to directions).

In a skillet, melt the margarine; remove from heat, add the flour and stir until smooth. Add the chicken bouillon, simmer for a few minutes until the sauce thickens. Set aside to cool. Add the egg substitute and the soy milk to the cooled sauce; heat and stir. Add the wine, mushrooms and chicken and heat gently, while stirring, for 10 minutes. Place the cooked spaghetti in a large baking dish and add the chicken-sauce mixture. Brown quickly in a broiler and serve hot.

NUTRIENTS, per serving:

Calories 362	Protein 39 gm	Carbohydrates 27 gm
Calcium 39 mg	Total fat 12 gm	Saturated fat 2 gm

EXCHANGES, per serving: 4½ meat; 2 bread

CHINESE CHICKEN   *4 servings*

½ *cup chicken bouillon*
¼ *cup soy sauce*
2 *tablespoons dry sherry*
1 *tablespoon cornstarch*
2 *tablespoons oil*
3 *cups chicken breasts, cut into 1 inch cubes*
½ *cup sliced celery*
1 *teaspoon minced garlic*
1 *cup sliced mushrooms*
1 *cup water chestnuts*
½ *cup bamboo shoots*

In a bowl, blend together bouillon, soy sauce, sherry and cornstarch until smooth. Set aside. In a non-stick skillet, heat oil and brown chicken. Remove from pan and keep warm. Add celery, garlic and mushrooms; stir for 2 minutes until mushrooms are slightly browned. Return chicken to pan, add water chestnuts and bamboo shoots, pour well-mixed sauce over all and cook for 2-3 minutes, until chicken is done and vegetables are tender. Serve with rice or noodles.

NUTRIENTS, per serving:

Calories 296	Protein 32 gm	Carbohydrates 7 gm
Calcium 29 mg	Total fat 12 gm	Saturated fat 3 gm

EXCHANGES, per serving: 4 meat; 1½ vegetable

STUFFED CORNISH HEN   *4 servings*

1 chopped small onion
¼ cup non-dairy margarine
1 cup soft milk-free bread cubes
2 stalks chopped celery
1 tablespoon chopped parsley
½ teaspoon poultry seasoning
pepper to taste
garlic powder to taste
2 Cornish hens (about 1-1½ pounds each)
poultry seasoning and paprika to taste
2 cups water
1 teaspoon chicken bouillon (dry)
1 tablespoon flour
½ cup mock sour cream or non-dairy sour cream

Saute onion in the margarine until transparent. Add bread cubes, celery, parsley, poultry seasoning and pepper; mix. Season cavity with garlic powder. Stuff each hen with about ½ cup of stuffing. Secure opening with skewer; fasten neck skin to back with skewer and tie legs together with string. Season hens with poultry seasoning and paprika. Place hens breast side up in shallow roasting pan; fashion an aluminum foil tent over birds. Roast hens in 350° oven for about ¾ to 1 hour. Remove foil and roast for additional 15 to 30 minutes, until brown. Cut hens along the backbone into 4 servings. Make a sauce by heating the water and chicken bouillon, then stirring in the flour until smooth; add the sour cream and stir. Pour over the hens.

NUTRIENTS, per serving:

Calories 320	Protein 29 gm	Carbohydrates 8 gm
Calcium 40 mg	Total fat 29 gm	Saturated fat 3 gm

EXCHANGES, per serving: 4 meat; ½ bread; 2 fat

CURRIED CHICKEN SALAD   *3 servings*

1 cup cooked chicken, diced
2 tablespoons chopped green onion
¼ cup chopped celery
1 teaspoon curry powder
2 tablespoons mock sour cream
2 tablespoons mayonnaise
1 teaspoon lemon juice

To the chicken in a blender, add the other ingredients and blend well until smooth. Serve chilled.

NUTRIENTS, per serving:

Calories 120	Protein 13 gm	Carbohydrates 1 gm
Calcium 9.3 mg	Total fat 6 gm	Saturated fat 1.5 gm

EXCHANGES, per serving: 2 meat

CHICKEN SANDWICH SPREAD   *6 servings*

2 cups cooked chicken, diced
¼ cup mayonnaise
2 tablespoons soy milk
½ cup chopped green pepper
¼ cup chopped red pepper
1 teaspoon onion powder
pepper to taste

Blend ingredients until smooth; use for sandwiches or canapes.

NUTRIENTS, per serving:

Calories 119	Protein 13 gm	Carbohydrates 1 gm
Calcium 9.5 mg	Total fat 6.5 gm	Saturated fat 1.5 gm

EXCHANGES, per serving: 2 meat

BEEF & LAMB

Beef, while an excellent source of protein, may contain more saturated fat than poultry. The recipes in this section, where possible, incorporate lean and less marbled cuts of such meats. To further reduce calories and fat intake, trim fat before cooking; and when sauteing, coat skillet with non-stick cooking spray.

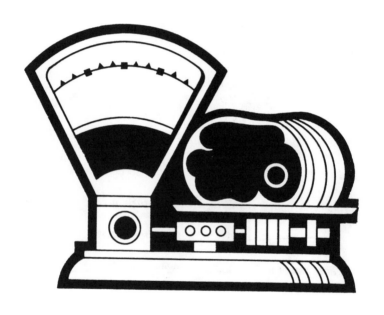

BEEF BURGUNDY   *6 servings*

1 small onion, sliced
2 tablespoons non-dairy margarine
2 pounds chuck, cut into 1 inch cubes
2 tablespoons flour
pepper to taste
1 cup beef bouillon
1 cup Burgundy wine
1 cup fresh mushrooms
1 cup mock sour cream (or non-dairy sour cream)

Saute onion in margarine; add meat and brown. Add flour and pepper and stir until smooth. Add 1 cup bouillon and the wine. Simmer 2½ hours. Add mushrooms and simmer another 30 minutes. If mixture needs thinning, add additional bouillon. Just before serving, stir in 1 cup of the sour cream. Serve with rice.

NUTRIENTS, per serving:

Calories 395	Protein 31 gm	Carbohydrates 4.5 gm
Calcium 57 mg	Total fat 25 gm	Saturated fat 9 gm

EXCHANGES, per serving: 4½ meat; ½ fat

MEAT LOAF I   *4 servings*

¼ cup mashed sweet potatoes
2 tablespoons chopped onion
1 tablespoon chopped parsley
¼ cup barbecue sauce
1 pound ground beef
½ cup corn flake crumbs
2 tablespoons egg substitute
pepper to taste

Blend sweet potato, onion and parsley flakes in barbecue sauce. Add to meat, crumbs, egg substitute and pepper. Mix thoroughly. Serve into 5 x 9 inch loaf pan. Bake at 350° for 45 minutes. Serve with tomato sauce on the side, and with green vegetables.

NUTRIENTS, per serving:

Calories 385	Protein 30 gm	Carbohydrates 17 gm
Calcium 44 mg	Total fat 21 gm	Saturated fat 8 gm

EXCHANGES, per serving: 4 meat; 1 bread

MEATLOAF II   *4 servings*

¼ cup egg substitute
1 pound ground beef
½ cup instant mashed potatoes
2 tablespoons chopped onion
½ teaspoon garlic powder
pepper to taste

Blend the egg substitute with the beef, then add remaining ingredients and mix thoroughly. Shape into a greased 5 x 9 inch loaf pan. Bake at 350° for 45 minutes. Serve with tomato sauce or mushroom sauce.

NUTRIENTS, per serving:

Calories 328	Protein 28 gm	Carbohydrates 5 gm
Calcium 26 mg	Total fat 21 gm	Saturated fat 8 gm

EXCHANGES, per serving: 4 meat

BEEF STROGANOFF I   *4 servings*

1 pound lean ground beef
1 teaspoon vegetable oil
2 cups sliced mushrooms
½ cup chopped onion
1 teaspoon minced garlic
2 tablespoons flour
1 cup chicken bouillon
½ cup dry red wine
1 cup non-pasteurized yogurt

In a non-stick pan, brown ground meat; add oil, mushrooms, onions and garlic and cook for 1-2 minutes, until mushrooms are browned. Stir in flour until well blended. Add chicken bouillon and wine; bring to boil, stirring constantly until thickened and smooth. Return meat to pan; simmer for 5 minutes. Stir in yogurt and serve over cooked noodles.

NUTRIENTS, per serving:

Calories 381	Protein 31 gm	Carbohydrates 9 gm
Calcium 125 mg	Total fat 22 gm	Saturated fat 8.5 gm

EXCHANGES, per serving: 4 meat; 2 vegetable; ½ fat

BEEF STROGANOFF II   *4 servings*

1 pound beef tenderloin, sliced into ½ inch strips
4 tablespoons non-dairy margarine
¼ cup sliced mushrooms
2 medium sliced onions
1 clove finely chopped garlic
½ cup water
1 teaspoon beef bouillon powder
¼ teaspoon pepper
1 cup Madeira wine
½ cup mock sour cream
½ teaspoon chopped parsley

Cut beef across grain into ½ inch strips. Heat 2 tablespoons margarine in a non-stick skillet until melted. Add mushrooms, onions and garlic. Cover and simmer, stirring occasionally, until onions are tender, 5 to 10 minutes. Remove vegetables and any liquid from skillet. Cook and stir beef in 2 tablespoons margarine over medium heat until brown, about 10 minutes. Add water, bouillon and pepper. Heat to boiling; reduce heat. Cover and simmer until beef is desired doneness, 10 to 15 minutes. Add vegetable mixture. Heat to boiling; reduce heat. Stir in wine, then the mock sour cream. Heat just until hot. Serve over noodles, garnished with parsley.

NUTRIENTS, per serving:

Calories 410	Protein 47.5 gm	Carbohydrates 5 gm
Calcium 53 mg	Total fat 17.5 gm	Saturated fat 3.6 gm

EXCHANGES, not applicable

SKEWERED BEEF AND TOFU   *6 servings*

¾ pound round steak, cut in 1 inch cubes
½ pound tofu, cut in 1½ inch cubes
¼ cup soy sauce
4 small whole onions
8 chunks canned pineapple, unsweetened
4 small cherry tomatoes
4 pieces of green pepper, 1½ inch square

Marinate the meat and tofu in the soy sauce for 1 hour. Drain the beef and tofu (save the sauce) and thread on skewers, along with the onions, pineapple, tomato and green peppers. Grill under the broiler, basting with the sauce, until the meat is tender, about 10 minutes.

NUTRIENTS, per serving:

Calories 265	Protein 21 gm	Carbohydrates 8 gm
Calcium 59 mg	Total fat 6 gm	Saturated fat 22 gm

EXCHANGES, per serving: 3 meat; ½ fruit

SWEDISH MEATBALLS   *8 servings*

1 pound ground beef
½ pound ground veal
1 egg
1 cup mashed potatoes
2 tablespoons grated onions
pepper to taste
¼ teaspoon nutmeg
1/8 teaspoon ginger
2 tablespoons oil
¼ cup water

Combine all ingredients except oil and water; form into 1 inch balls. Heat oil in a large non-stick skillet; brown meatballs over low heat, shaking pan occasionally to brown all sides. Add ¼ cup water, cover and simmer 20 minutes. Serve with mustard or barbecue sauce.

NUTRIENTS, per serving:

Calories 301	Protein 20 gm	Carbohydrates 4.5 gm
Calcium 20 mg	Total fat 23 gm	Saturated fat 8 gm

EXCHANGES, per serving: 3 meat; 2 fat

SZECHUAN PEPPERED BEEF   *4 servings*

1 pound flank steak, cut into 2 inch by ¼ inch slices
2 slices ginger root
1½ tablespoons soy sauce
1½ tablespoons hoisin sauce
1 tablespoon Worcestershire sauce
pepper to taste
3 tablespoons vegetable oil
1 green pepper, cut into 1 inch squares

Marinate the beef with the ginger root, soy, hoisin and Worcestershire sauces; add pepper. Keep beef covered with this mixture for about 1 hour, turning occasionally. Heat oil in skillet; when hot, add the meat from marinade and saute for 2 minutes, then turn over and saute for another minute; add green pepper; pour in saved marinade and stir-fry for 30 seconds. Serve hot over rice.

NUTRIENTS, per serving:

Calories 361	Protein 28.5 gm	Carbohydrates 2 gm
Calcium 18 mg	Total fat 27.5 gm	Saturated fat 8 gm

EXCHANGES, per serving: 4 meat; 1½ fat

GOULASH

6 servings

2 tablespoons vegetable oil
1½ pounds round steak, cut in 1 inch cubes
2 medium onions, chopped
1 clove garlic, chopped
3 cups water
2 tablespoons paprika
2 teaspoons chicken bouillon powder
pepper to taste
¼ cup cold water
2 tablespoons cornstarch
½ cup mock sour cream or non-dairy sour cream

Heat oil in large non-stick skillet, add beef; cook in hot oil until brown; drain on paper towels. Cook and stir onions and garlic in skillet until onions are tender; drain fat. Add beef, 3 cups water, paprika, bouillon powder and pepper. Heat to boiling; reduce heat, cover and simmer until beef is tender, about 1½ hours. Stir ¼ cup water with the cornstarch until smooth, then stir into beef mixture. Heat to boiling, stirring constantly for 1 minute; reduce heat. Stir in sour cream; heat until hot. Serve over cooked noodles.

NUTRIENTS, per serving:

Calories 247	Protein 27 gm	Carbohydrates 6 gm
Calcium 28 mg	Total fat 12 gm	Saturated fat 3 gm

EXCHANGES, per serving: 3½ meat; 1 vegetable

BRAISED BEEF   *6 servings*

1 ½ pounds round steak
3 tablespoons flour
2 tablespoons vegetable oil
2 cups beef bouillon
3 carrots, sliced
2 medium onions, sliced
pepper to taste
¼ teaspoons dried thyme leaves
½ cup mock sour cream

Cut beef into 1 inch cubes. Sprinkle one side of beef with half the flour and pound in; turn beef; pound in remaining flour. Heat oil in non-stick skillet until hot. Brown on both sides, about 15 minutes; drain. Add bouillon and heat to boiling. Reduce heat, cover and simmer 15 minutes. Add carrots and onions. Sprinkle with pepper and thyme. Cover and simmer until beef and vegetables are tender, 40 to 60 minutes. Stir in mock sour cream. Serve over broad noodles.

NUTRIENTS, per serving::

Calories 202	Protein 26.5 gm	Carbohydrates 5 gm
Calcium 51 mg	Total fat 8 gm	Saturated fat 2.8 gm

EXCHANGES, per serving: 3½ meat; 1 vegetable

MEAT CASSEROLE

6 servings

1 pound ground beef
1 chopped onion
½ teaspoon minced garlic
½ teaspoon dried basil
½ teaspoon dried oregano
1 cup tomato sauce
6 ounces of noodles, cooked according to package directions
¼ cup mock sour cream

Brown ground meat slowly in a non-stick skillet; add onion and garlic and cook for 2 minutes. Stir in spices and tomato sauce and bring to boil; reduce heat and simmer until sauce is thick. Place noodles in lightly greased rectangular baking dish; cover with meat mixture. Bake at 350° for 45 minutes; stir in the mock sour cream before serving.

NUTRIENTS, per serving:

Calories 346	Protein 24.5 gm	Carbohydrates 26 gm
Calcium 41.5 mg	Total fat 15 gm	Saturated fat 5 gm

EXCHANGES, per serving: 2½ meat; 1½ bread; ½ fat; ½ vegetable

WIENER SCHNITZEL

4 servings

2 veal cutlets cut in half and pounded to ¼ inch thickness
(total weight about 2 pounds)
2 tablespoons flour
½ cup soy milk
2 tablespoons egg substitute
2 tablespoons grated Parmesan cheese substitute
2 tablespoons non-dairy margarine
pepper to taste

Dust the cutlets with the flour; blend soy milk with egg substitute and cheese substitute. Coat cutlets with the mixture and saute in skillet in the melted margarine, turning to brown both sides. Cover skillet and cook for additional 10 minutes. Season. Serve hot, garnished with lemon slices.

<u>NUTRIENTS</u>, per serving:

Calories 290	Protein 26 gm	Carbohydrates 1 gm
Calcium 27 mg	Total fat 19 gm	Saturated fat 6 gm

<u>EXCHANGES</u>, per serving: 4 meat

VEAL IN SOUR CREAM
6 servings

12 slices of veal (total weight about 1½ pounds)
3 tablespoons flour
3 tablespoons non-dairy margarine
½ cup chopped onions
1 cup sliced mushrooms
¼ cup cognac
½ cup mock sour cream
6 canned apricot halves

Dust the dry veal slices with flour and saute in a non-stick skillet, a few at a time in hot margarine until brown on each side (2-4 minutes total time); remove to a dish. When all the slices have been sauteed, add the onions to the skillet and cook until transparent; then add the mushrooms and cook for an additional 10 minutes, until tender. Remove from heat, add the cognac slowly, then stir in the sour cream substitute. Add the veal slices to this sauce and heat for ½ minute. Garnish with apricot halves before serving.

NUTRIENTS, per serving:

| Calories 305 | Protein 25 gm | Carbohydrates 9 gm |
| Calcium 52 mg | Total fat 16 gm | Saturated fat 5 gm |

EXCHANGES, per serving: 3 meat; ½ bread

VEAL RIBS IN CREAM AND SAGE SAUCE   *6 servings*

2 tablespoons non-dairy margarine
4 pounds of veal ribs
1 cup chopped onions
1 tablespoon flour
1 cup water
1 tablespoon chopped garlic
½ cup soy milk
1 tablespoon ground sage
pepper to taste

Melt the margarine in a non-stick skillet and brown the veal ribs on all sides. Remove the ribs; discard most of the fat from the skillet. Saute the onions until soft. Add the flour, then the water; bring to a boil, stirring constantly. Add the ribs and the garlic; cover. Cook for 1 hour, until tender. Add the soy milk; bring to a boil; add the sage and pepper. Serve with rice.

NUTRIENTS, per serving:

| Calories 237 | Protein 24 gm | Carbohydrates 2.8 gm |
| Calcium 22.6 mg | Total fat 13.6 gm | Saturated fat 4.6 gm |

EXCHANGES, per serving: 3½ meat

BAKED VEAL CUTLETS

6 servings

1½ pound veal cutlets
½ cup soy milk
1 cup bran flakes, crushed
1 tablespoon chopped parsley
1 teaspoon oregano
2 teaspoons vegetable oil

Pound the veal until it is about ¼ inch thick. Dip each cutlet in the milk, then into a mixture of the bran flakes, parsley and oregano. Arrange the cutlets in a lightly oiled baking pan and bake at 350° for 45 minutes. Serve with broccoli.

NUTRIENTS, per serving:

Calories 352	Protein 28 gm	Carbohydrates 25 gm
Calcium 40 mg	Total fat 14 gm	Saturated fat 4 gm

EXCHANGES, per serving: 3 meat; 1½ bread

VEAL WITH CHEESE

4 servings

1 tablespoon non-dairy margarine
8 slices veal (12 ounces), pounded flat
2 slices non-dairy Mozzarella cheese
½ pound canned tomatoes
pepper to taste
1 teaspoon oregano
½ teaspoon chopped parsley

Melt margarine in a non-stick skillet; saute both sides of the veal. Transfer to a shallow baking pan coated with non-stick cooking spray; place half a slice of cheese on each piece of veal. In a separate bowl, finely chop the tomatoes; add spices; mix well. Add this sauce to the veal. Bake in a preheated 450° oven for 25 minutes, until tender. Garnish with parsley before serving.

NUTRIENTS, per serving:

Calories 250	Protein 28 gm	Carbohydrates 3.5 gm
Calcium 200 mg	Total fat 18 gm	Saturated fat 3 gm

EXCHANGES, per serving: 4 meat

VEAL PARMESAN (CHEESELESS)   *4 servings*

½ cup flour
pepper to taste
¼ teaspoon paprika
4 veal chops
¼ cup egg substitute
2 tablespoons vegetable oil
8 thin slices tomatoes
¼ cup minced onions
½ cup sliced mushrooms
¼ cup mayonnaise

Blend the first three ingredients. Dredge the veal chops in the seasoned flour, dip in the egg, and then into the flour again. Saute the veal in the heated oil, in a non-stick skillet, until brown on both sides. Place in a greased baking pan. Top with tomato slices. In the skillet used for the veal, saute the onions until transparent; stir in the mushrooms and continue cooking for 1 minute. Cool; blend in the mayonnaise and pour this mixture over the veal. Bake at 375° until brown, about 30 minutes; drain excess oil before serving.

NUTRIENTS, per serving:

Calories 340	Protein 27 gm	Carbohydrates 4.5 gm
Calcium 34 mg	Total fat 22 gm	Saturated fat 6 gm

EXCHANGES, 4 meat; ½ fat

VEAL STEW   *12 servings*

3 pounds veal shoulder, cut into 1 inch cubes
3 cups beef bouillon
½ cup celery, cut into 1 inch pieces
1 large onion, cut into quarters
1 large carrot, cut in 1 inch slices
¼ cup flour
¼ cup non-dairy margarine
1 cup soy milk
2 teaspoons lemon juice
¼ teaspoon chopped parsley

In large pot, add the veal and the beef bouillon, celery, onion and carrot and cook for 1½ hours. Blend the flour and margarine in a small pan, while heating and stirring until smooth, then add to the veal mixture and simmer for 10 minutes. Add the milk, stirring for a few seconds, then add the lemon juice. Sprinkle with parsley before serving.

NUTRIENTS, per serving:

Calories 316	Protein 24 gm	Carbohydrates 3 gm
Calcium 20 mg	Total fat 22 gm	Saturated fat 8 gm

EXCHANGES, per serving: 3½ meat; 1 fat

LAMB SOUVLAKI

8 servings

1 pound ground lamb
1 chopped onion
½ teaspoon minced garlic
2 cups stewed tomatoes
1½ cups chicken bouillon
¼ teaspoon oregano
1 cup brown rice, uncooked
4 cups fresh chopped lettuce
4 pita breads, cut in half to make pockets
¼ cup mock sour cream

Heat lamb in a large skillet coated with non-stick spray, slowly, until lightly browned on all sides; add onion and garlic and cook until limp. Stir in tomatoes, bouillon and oregano and bring to a boil. Add brown rice, cover and simmer for 45 minutes or until rice is tender. Stir lettuce into lamb/rice mixture just before serving and heat through. Remove from heat, place into pita pockets; add mock sour cream before serving.

NUTRIENTS, per serving::

Calories 340	Protein 17.6 gm	Carbohydrates 27 gm
Calcium 64 mg	Total fat 17 gm	Saturated fat 7 gm

EXCHANGES, per serving: 1½ meat; 1½ bread; 2 fat

LAMB SAUTEED IN CREAM

4 servings

1 pound lamb, cut into 1 inch cubes
1 tablespoon non-dairy margarine
¼ cup lactose-reduced milk
½ teaspoon dried parsley

In a non-stick pan, saute the lamb in the margarine, until brown on all sides; remove from pan to serving platter. Add the milk to the juices in the pan, simmer and reduce to half the original volume. Pour over lamb pieces; garnish with parsley. Serve with noodles and a green vegetable.

NUTRIENTS, per serving::

| Calories 271 | Protein 24 gm | Carbohydrates 1 gm |
| Calcium 28 mg | Total fat 19 gm | Saturated fat 7 gm |

EXCHANGES, per serving: 3½ meat

DESSERTS

A bonus from learning to cook with non-dairy foods is the surprising number of desserts -- including chocolate cakes and ice creams -- that can be made without milk products. But it is wise, in general, to reduce sugar intake; people with diabetes especially should note that foods high in sugar include frosted cakes, pies, syrups and honey.

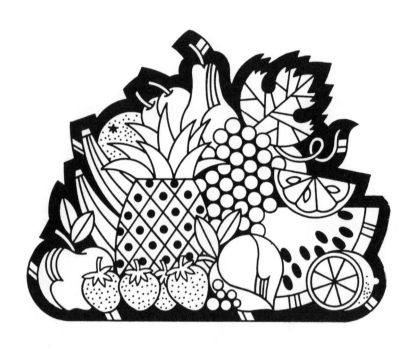

STEWED FIGS

6 servings

1 pound dried figs
1 cup dry white wine
1 cup water
¼ cup sugar
1 tablespoon lemon juice
1/8 teaspoon cinnamon

Soak the figs in the wine and water overnight; add the sugar and juice and simmer for 15 minutes, or until tender. Add cinnamon. Serve cold.

NUTRIENTS, per serving:

Calories 154	Protein 1 gm	Carbohydrates 34 gm
Calcium 56 mg	Total fat 0.6 gm	Saturated fat 0.1 gm

EXCHANGES, not applicable

PRUNE WHIP

8 servings

1 pound of canned prune filling
½ cup sugar
2 cups non-dairy whipped topping

Blend the prune filling with the sugar; fold in 1 cup of the whipped topping and serve with the remaining topping as garnish.

NUTRIENTS, per serving:

Calories 186	Protein 1 gm	Carbohydrates 42 gm
Calcium 21.5 mg	Total fat 4.2 gm	Saturated fat 0.0 gm

EXCHANGES, not applicable

FRUIT CRISP   *10 servings*

¾ cup oats, uncooked
½ cup brown sugar
¾ teaspoon cinnamon
4 teaspoon non-dairy margarine, melted
¼ cup orange juice
2 tablespoons flour
4 cups apples, peeled and sliced thin
2 cups dried apricots, chopped

Blend oats, ¼ cup sugar, ¼ teaspoon cinnamon and margarine; set aside. In an 8 inch glass baking dish, thoroughly blend the remaining ingredients. Top this fruit mixture with the reserved oat blend. Bake for 45 minutes in a 350° preheated oven. Spoon (hot or cold) into dessert dishes.

NUTRIENTS, per serving:

Calories 189	Protein 2.4 gm	Carbohydrates 30 gm
Calcium 26 mg	Total fat 5.5 gm	Saturated fat 0.8 gm

EXCHANGES, not applicable

PEANUT BUTTER COOKIES   *24 cookies*

½ cup non-dairy margarine
½ cup peanut butter
½ cup sugar
½ cup firmly packed brown sugar
1 egg
1¼ cups all purpose flour
1 teaspoon baking powder
1 teaspoon baking soda

Blend together margarine, peanut butter, sugars and egg. Sift together dry ingredients; add to creamed mixture. Beat well. Roll into 1 inch balls. Place 3 inches apart on cookie sheet and flatten with a fork, making a crosshatch pattern. Bak in a 325° preheated oven for 15-18 minutes, until cookies are set.

NUTRIENTS, per cookie:

Calories 105	Protein 2 gm	Carbohydrates 10 gm
Calcium 12 mg	Total fat 6.8 gm	Saturated fat 4 gm

EXCHANGES, not applicable

DATE-NUT COOKIES   *24 cookies*

1 egg
½ cup egg substitute
2 cups brown sugar
1 teaspoon vanilla extract
¾ cup chunky peanut butter
½ cup chopped dates

Beat the eggs and egg substitute in a mixing bowl until thick; stir in sugar and vanilla. Add peanut butter and dates; mix well; chill 2 hours. Drop by teaspoonfuls onto a greased cookie sheet; flatten with a fork. Bake in a preheated 300° oven until cookies are lightly browned, about 25 minutes.

NUTRIENTS, per cookie:

Calories 154	Protein 1 gm	Carbohydrates 34 gm
Calcium 56 mg	Total fat 0.6 gm	Saturated fat 0.1 gm

EXCHANGES, not applicable

CHOCOLATE CHIP COOKIES   *24 cookies*

1 cup all-purpose flour
1 teaspoon baking soda
½ cup non-dairy margarine
½ cup sugar
½ cup firmly packed brown sugar
1 teaspoon vanilla extract
2 eggs
6 ounces milk-free chocolate chips
½ cup chopped walnuts

Sift together flour and baking soda. Separately, cream margarine, sugars, vanilla and eggs until light and fluffy. Add dry ingredients and mix well. Stir in chocolate chips and nuts. Drop by teaspoon 2″ apart on cookie sheet. Bake in a preheated 325° oven for 15-18 minutes, until lightly browned.

NUTRIENTS, per cookie:

Calories 152	Protein 2.5 gm	Carbohydrates 16 gm
Calcium 9 mg	Total fat 9.5 gm	Saturated fat 2 gm

EXCHANGES, not applicable

OATMEAL COOKIES   *48 cookies*

½ cup non-dairy margarine
1 cup firmly packed brown sugar
1 cup sugar
1 teaspoon vanilla extract
1 cup flour
4 teaspoons baking powder
¾ cup orange juice
3 cups oatmeal
½ cup chopped walnuts

Blend margarine, sugars and vanilla. Sift together flour and baking powder, then add to blended mixture, while alternately adding the orange juice. Add oatmeal and nuts; mix well. Drop by teaspoon on greased cookie sheet. Bake in preheated 350° oven for 10 minutes.

NUTRIENTS, per cookie:

Calories 85	Protein 1.3 gm	Carbohydrates 14 gm
Calcium 8.4 mg	Total fat 3 gm	Saturated fat 0.4 gm

EXCHANGES, not applicable

FUDGE BROWNIES   *16 servings*

½ cup non-dairy margarine
2 ounces unsweetened chocolate
1 cup flour
½ teaspoon baking powder
1 cup sugar
2 eggs
1 teaspoon vanilla extract
½ cup chopped walnuts

Melt margarine and chocolate over low heat. Sift together dry ingredients, stir into chocolate mixture and cool slightly. Add eggs, vanilla and nuts. Beat until smooth. Pour into a 9 inch square baking pan; bake in a 325° preheated oven for 20 minutes. Cool and cut into squares.

NUTRIENTS, per serving:

Calories 167	Protein 3.6 gm	Carbohydrates 19 gm
Calcium 13.5 mg	Total fat 12 gm	Saturated fat 2 gm

EXCHANGES, not applicable

CHOCOLATE TOFU BROWNIES   *12 servings*

1¼ cups flour
½ teaspoon baking soda
½ cup non-dairy margarine
¾ cup sugar
2 tablespoons vegetable oil
10 ounces tofu, drained and cut into 1 inch cubes
½ cup cocoa powder
2 teaspoons vanilla extract
¼ cup chopped walnuts

Sift the flour and the baking soda together; set aside. In a food processor, add the margarine, sugar and oil and blend until fluffy (1-2 minutes); add the tofu and blend an additional 2 minutes; add the cocoa and vanilla and blend for 1 minute. Add the flour-baking soda mixture slowly, blending after each addition; stir in the nuts. Pour this batter into a greased 9 inch square baking pan; bake in a preheated 450° oven for 20-30 minutes.

NUTRIENTS, per serving:

Calories 245	Protein 5 gm	Carbohydrates 19 gm
Calcium 41 mg	Total fat 4 gm	Saturated fat 0.4 gm

EXCHANGES, not applicable

MACROONS   *18 cookies*

1 cup finely ground almonds
¾ cup sugar
2 egg whites
2 tablespoons cornstarch
2 teaspoons water

Combine ground almonds and sugar. Add unbeaten egg whites, reserving about 1 tablespoon to brush on top of macroons. Blend for 1 minute, then add cornstarch and water, stirring well after each addition. Drop batter, by teaspoonfuls, 3 inches apart onto foil-covered cookie sheet. Brush cookies with remaining egg white, then bake in 375° oven 15 minutes. Cool for 3-4 minutes, then remove from foil.

NUTRIENTS, per serving:

Calories 111	Protein 7.5 gm	Carbohydrates 12 gm
Calcium 207 mg	Total fat 3 gm	Saturated fat 1.6 gm

EXCHANGES, not applicable

CHEESECAKE   *8 servings*

Cheese obtained from filtering 32 ounces of non-pasteurized yogurt
1 tablespoon cornstarch
1 teaspoon lemon juice
2 tablespoons sugar
2 teaspoons vanilla extract
2 eggs, beaten

Place the yogurt cheese in a bowl; add the cornstarch, lemon juice, sugar and vanilla; blend well. Stir in the eggs. Pour the mixture into a 9 inch greased pie pan and bake in a preheated 325° oven for about 25 minutes (the center of the pie should be set at this time). Serve chilled; garnish with sliced berries.

NUTRIENTS, per serving:

Calories 108	Protein 7.5 gm	Carbohydrates 12 gm
Calcium 207 mg	Total fat 3 gm	Saturated fat 1.6 gm

EXCHANGES, not applicable

FUDGE CAKE   *16 servings*

½ cup flour
¼ cup cocoa powder
2 teaspoons baking powder
1 teaspoon baking soda
1 teaspoon vanilla extract
½ cup non-dairy margarine
1 cup cold water

Frosting

¼ cup non-dairy margarine
1 cup confectioners sugar
¼ cup cocoa
¼ cup strong coffee

Sift the dry ingredients together in a mixing bowl. Add the remaining ingredients. Beat at medium speed for 3 minutes until batter is very smooth. Pour into greased 9 x 5 inch loaf pan; bake at 325° for 40 minutes.

Frosting: Cream margarine; blend in sifted sugar and sifted cocoa; add coffee gradually, stirring until spreadable consistency is obtained. Ice the cake when cool.

NUTRIENTS, per serving:

Calories 189	Protein 1 gm	Carbohydrates 19 gm
Calcium 10 mg	Total fat 14 gm	Saturated fat 3.8 gm

EXCHANGES, not applicable

TOFU CHEESECAKE I

12 servings

2 eggs
2 egg whites
8 ounces tofu, squeezed dry
¼ cup maple syrup
2 tablespoons lemon juice
2 teaspoons vanilla extract
4 ounces non-dairy cream cheese
2 cups sliced strawberries

Graham Cracker Crust

1 cup finely ground graham cracker crumbs
¼ cup non-dairy margarine, melted
1 teaspoon sugar

Whip the eggs in a processor for a few seconds. Add the tofu in small pieces, then add the maple syrup, lemon juice and vanilla extract. Blend the mixture until smooth. Add the cheese substitute, a little at a time; blend until smooth. Pour the filling into the prepared crust (made by blending the cracker crumbs, margarine and sugar, then pressing the mixture into a 9 inch pie pan). Bake in a preheated 325° oven for 40 minutes. Cool for a few minutes, then cover with the berries. Chill before serving.

NUTRIENTS, per serving:

Calories 173	Protein 4.5 gm	Carbohydrates 18 gm
Calcium 49.5 mg	Total fat 9.5 gm	Saturated fat 2.5 gm

EXCHANGES, not applicable

TOFU CHEESECAKE II   *12 servings*

20 ounces tofu, pressed dry
½ cup honey
3 tablespoons orange juice
2 teaspoons vanilla extract
2 tablespoons vegetable oil
2 tablespoons grated orange peel
9 inch graham cracker crust, (see previous recipe)

Blend the first six ingredients in a mixer for 30-40 seconds, until smooth. Pour into the 9 inch graham cracker crust and bake in a preheated 350° oven for 1 hour. Serve well chilled, topped with sliced strawberries.

<u>NUTRIENTS</u>, per serving:

Calories 177	Protein 4 gm	Carbohydrates 24 gm
Calcium 59 mg	Total fat 22 gm	Saturated fat 0.8 gm

<u>EXCHANGES</u>, per serving: not applicable

LEMON SPONGE CAKE   *10 servings*

4 egg yolks
¾ cup sugar
2 tablespoons lemon juice
1 lemon rind, grated
½ cup flour
1 teaspoon baking powder
4 egg whites
½ teaspoon cream of tartar

In a mixer, beat egg yolks, sugar, lemon juice and rind at medium speed, until thick and lemon colored (at least 10 minutes). Sift together dry ingredients, add to egg yolk mixture and beat at low speed for 2 minutes. In a separate bowl, beat egg whites and cream of tartar until stiff peaks are formed. Fold into egg yolk mixture. Pour batter into ungreased 10 inch tube pan. Bake in a preheated 325° oven for 40 to 45 minutes, until gold. Cool before serving.

NUTRIENTS, per serving:

Calories 209	Protein 3 gm	Carbohydrates 19 gm
Calcium 12 mg	Total fat 2 gm	Saturated fat 0.7 gm

EXCHANGES, not applicable

ANGEL FOOD CAKE   *10 servings*

12 egg whites
¼ teaspoon salt
1 teaspoon cream of tartar
1¼ cups sugar
1 cup confectioners' sugar
1¼ cups flour
1 tablespoon lemon juice

Be sure egg whites are at room temperature; add salt and beat until foamy. Add cream of tartar and beat until soft peaks form. Sift together sugar, confectioners' sugar, and flour; fold into egg whites. Fold in lemon juice, then pour into an ungreased 10 inch tube pan and bake in a 375° preheated oven for 45 minutes; cool before removing from pan. Note: Chocolate angel food cake may be prepared by replacing ¼ cup of the flour with ¼ cup cocoa powder.

NUTRIENTS, per serving:

Calories 209   Protein 5.4 gm   Carbohydrates 47 gm
Calcium 7 mg   Total fat 0.1 gm   Saturated fat 0.0 gm

EXCHANGES, not applicable

COFFEE CAKE   *16 servings*

½ cup non-dairy margarine, softened
2 cups sugar (save 1 tablespoon for topping)
2 eggs
½ cup egg substitute
3 cups flour
3 teaspoons baking powder
1 cup orange juice
2 ounces bittersweet chocolate bits
2 teaspoons cinnamon

Blend the first four ingredients. Sift the flour and baking powder together; alternately add the flour mixture and the juice to the margarine-sugar blend. Stir in the chocolate and pour the batter into a 9 x 13 inch cake pan. Top with cinnamon and sugar. Bake in a 350° preheated oven for 1 hour. Serve warm or cold.

NUTRIENTS, per serving:

Calories 263   Protein 4 gm   Carbohydrates 44 gm
Calcium 27 mg   Total fat 8 gm   Saturated fat 2 gm

EXCHANGES, not applicable

BANANA CAKE

8 servings

2 cups all purpose flour
3 teaspoons baking powder
1 teaspoon baking soda
1 cup sugar
2 eggs
¼ cup egg substitute
½ cup vegetable oil
1 teaspoon vanilla extract
1½ cups mashed bananas

Sift together dry ingredients. Add remaining ingredients; beat until smooth. Pour into an 8″ square greased pan and bake in a 350° preheated oven for 25 minutes. Cool before serving.

NUTRIENTS, per serving:

Calories 381	Protein 5.8 gm	Carbohydrates 56 gm
Calcium 19 mg	Total fat 16 gm	Saturated fat 2.6 gm

EXCHANGES, not applicable

CHOCOLATE FROSTING

10 servings
Frosts a 9 inch cake

½ cup non-dairy margarine softened
2 cups confectioners sugar
½ cup egg substitute
½ cup cocoa powder

Cream margarine and sifted sugar until fluffy. Add egg substitute, beat, then beat in sifted cocoa. If frosting is too thick, add warm water by teaspoonfuls until frosting is spreadable.

NUTRIENTS, per serving:

Calories 217	Protein 2.4 gm	Carbohydrates 26 gm
Calcium 16 mg	Total fat 13 gm	Saturated fat 3 gm

EXCHANGES, not applicable

CHOCOLATE FUDGE   *16 pieces*

1¼ cups soy milk
4 ounces unsweetened chocolate
4 cups granulated sugar
2 tablespoons corn syrup
1 tablespoon non-dairy margarine
2 teaspoons vanilla extract

Heat the milk in a saucepan, add chocolate and cook together until chocolate melts.   Add the sugar and corn syrup, stirring until everything is dissolved; continue heating until the mixture reaches soft ball stage. Remove from heat, add the margarine and vanilla and let cool to 100°. Beat well for about 15 seconds. Pour into greased 8 inch square pan; cool, then cut into squares.

NUTRIENTS, per piece:

Calories 247	Protein 1.4 gm	Carbohydrates 52 gm
Calcium 10 mg	Total fat 4.7 gm	Saturated fat 2 gm

EXCHANGES, not applicable

PIE PASTRY
2 crusts, 9-inch

2 cups flour
2/3 cup non-dairy margarine
4-5 tablespoons cold water

Mix flour and margarine together until a coarse mixture is obtained. Slowly add water, 1 tablespoon at a time, blending in thoroughly. Refrigerate at least one hour, then divide the dough into two crusts, rolling each on a floured board. Line two 9 inch pie pans, prick the pie shell with a fork and bake in a preheated 425° oven for 8 minutes.
Note: Nutrient values for 1 crust: 450 calories; 12 gm protein; 90 gm carbohydrates; 57 gm fat. These nutrient values are incorporated in specific pie recipes.

FRUIT MOUSSE
6 servings

2 ripe bananas
1 whole orange, peeled
1 whole kiwi, peeled
1 cup frozen strawberries
1 cup non-pasteurized yogurt
3 tablespoons sugar
1 envelope gelatin
½ cup water

Blend all fruits together in blender or food processor. Add yogurt and sugar; blend until smooth. Soften gelatin in ¼ cup cold water, then add ¼ cup boiling water to dissolve. Add the gelatin mixture to fruit and blend well. Pour into parfait dishes; chill before serving.

NUTRIENTS, per serving:

Calories 105	Protein 3 gm	Carbohydrates 23 gm
Calcium 82 mg	Total fat 1.0 gm	Saturated fat 0.5 gm

EXCHANGES, not applicable

CHOCOLATE MOUSSE   *8 servings*

1 tablespoon instant coffee
1 tablespoon boiling water
4 ounces semi-sweet chocolate
2 eggs, separated, plus 1 egg white
4 tablespoons sugar
2 tablespoons brandy

Dissolve coffee in boiling water, add chocolate and melt slowly over very low heat. Let cool. Beat the three egg whites until stiff; set aside. In a separate bowl, beat the 2 egg yolks until thick; add sugar and beat until well dissolved. Pour cooled chocolate/coffee mixture and brandy into egg yolks and stir well. Fold this mixture gently into the beaten egg whites. Pour into parfait dishes; serve chilled.

NUTRIENTS, per serving:

Calories 114	Protein 2 gm	Carbohydrates 14 gm
Calcium 11 mg	Total fat 6 gm	Saturated fat 3 gm

EXCHANGES, not applicable

PUMPKIN PIE   *8 servings*

2 cups canned pumpkin
2/3 cups firmly packed brown sugar
1½ cups water
6 tablespoons cornstarch
1 tablespoon pumpkin pie spice
1 unbaked pie crust, 9 inch
½ cup brown sugar

Combine all ingredients for pie filling in sauce pan; cook over low heat until mixture begins to thicken, stirring constantly. Pour into 9 inch pie crust; bake in a 375° oven for 30 minutes. Sprinkle brown sugar on top of pie; bake for additional 5 minutes.

NUTRIENTS, per cookie:

Calories 366	Protein 3.6 gm	Carbohydrates 56 gm
Calcium 46 mg	Total fat 15 gm	Saturated fat 3 gm

EXCHANGES, not applicable

LEMON PIE   *8 servings*

1 cup sugar
¼ cup cornstarch
1 cup water
2 tablespoons grated lemon rind
½ cup lemon juice
2 tablespoons non-dairy margarine
1 baked pie crust, 9 inch

Mix sugar and cornstarch in sauce pan; stir water in gradually. Cook over medium heat while stirring until mixture thickens and boils. When mixture is clear, add lemon rind, juice and margarine; remove from heat and chill. Spoon into 9 inch baked pie crust; serve cold.

NUTRIENTS, per cookie:

Calories 363	Protein 3 gm	Carbohydrates 50 gm
Calcium 11 mg	Total fat 17 gm	Saturated fat 3 gm

EXCHANGES, not applicable

APRICOT CREAM PIE   *8 servings*

1 envelope unflavored gelatin
¼ cup cold water
1 cup apricot pulp (from 6 pureed dried apricots)
½ cup apricot nectar
1 tablespoon lemon juice
1/3 cup sugar
1 cup whipped non-dairy topping
1 baked pie crust, 9 inch

Soften gelatin in cold water; heat together apricot pulp and nectar,
lemon juice and sugar. Add softened gelatin and stir until dissolved.
Chill until partially set, then whip until fluffy. Fold in whipped
topping. Pour into baked 9 inch pie crust; serve chilled.

NUTRIENTS, per serving:

Calories 349	Protein 4.5 gm	Carbohydrates 47 gm
Calcium 15 mg	Total fat 17 gm	Saturated fat 5 gm

EXCHANGES, not applicable

BANANA CREAM PIE   *8 servings*

6 ounces tofu
1 pound bananas (save 1 banana)
2 tablespoons vegetable oil
2 tablespoons honey
1 tablespoon soy milk
1 teaspoon lemon juice
½ teaspoon vanilla extract
¼ teaspoon cinnamon
1 baked pie crust, 9 inch

Blend the first eight ingredients until smooth. Layer saved banana slices on the bottom of the pie shell, then pour in the filling. Decorate the top of the pie with a few banana slices which have been dipped in lemon juice to prevent browning. Serve chilled.

NUTRIENTS, per serving:

Calories 333   Protein 5 gm   Carbohydrates 38 gm
Calcium 33 mg   Total fat 19 gm   Saturated fat 3.4 gm

EXCHANGES, not applicable

CHOCOLATE CREAM PIE   *8 servings*

1 envelope unflavored gelatin
¼ cup cold water
3 eggs, separated
½ cup sugar
1 teaspoon vanilla extract
2 tablespoons cognac
2 tablespoons non-dairy margarine
6 tablespoons cocoa powder
½ cup water
½ cup sugar
1 graham cracker crust, 9 inch (see page 187)

Soften gelatin in ¼ cup cold water and set aside. Beat egg yolks until thick; beat in ½ cup sugar, vanilla and cognac. In a small pan, over very low heat, melt margarine and add cocoa and ½ cup water; stir until well blended. Add softened gelatin, stirring until dissolved. Beat chocolate mixture into egg yolks; chill until almost set. Beat room-temperature egg whites until stiff; gradually add ½ cup sugar, while beating. Fold chocolate mixture into egg whites. Pour cooled filling into 9 inch graham cracker crust; serve chilled.

NUTRIENTS, per serving:

Calories 326   Protein 5 gm   Carbohydrates 41 gm
Calcium 26 mg   Total fat 18 gm   Saturated fat 4 gm

EXCHANGES, not applicable

LIME SHERBET   *6 servings*

2 egg whites
¼ cup sugar
1 cup light corn syrup
2 cups soy milk
3 lime rinds, grated
¾ cup lime juice

Beat the egg whites until stiff; continue to beat, while adding the remaining ingredients. Pour the blend into a freezer tray and freeze until firm; transfer sherbet into a mixing bowl and beat until creamy. Return to freezer tray and freeze until firm.

NUTRIENTS, per serving:

Calories 235   Protein 4 gm   Carbohydrates 52 gm
Calcium 22 mg   Total fat 1.3 gm   Saturated fat 0.0 gm

EXCHANGES, not applicable

APRICOT SHERBET   *6 servings*

1 envelope unflavored gelatin
½ cup cold water
3 cups apricot nectar
¾ cup light corn syrup
¼ cup lemon juice

Sprinkle gelatin on water in sauce pan. Place over low heat, stirring constantly, until gelatin is dissolved. Stir in remaining ingredients. Pour into two refrigerator trays and freeze until firm (1 hour). Place in chilled bowl and beat until light and creamy. Return to trays and freeze for several hours until firm.

NUTRIENTS, per serving:

Calories 196	Protein 1 gm	Carbohydrates 48 gm
Calcium 8.5 mg	Total fat 0.1 gm	Saturated fat 0.0 gm

EXCHANGES, not applicable

ORANGE ICE   *8 servings*

2 cups sugar
4 cups water
2 cups orange juice
¼ cup lemon juice
2 orange rinds, grated

Boil sugar and water 5 minutes. Add fruit juices and grated rind. Cool and strain. Freeze in refrigerator trays.

Calories 219	Protein 0.4 gm	Carbohydrates 54.5 gm
Calcium 6.7 mg	Total fat 0.1 gm	Saturated fat 0.0 gm

EXCHANGES, not applicable

CHOCOLATE ICE CREAM   *6 servings*

6 eggs whites
¾ cup sugar
2 cups non-dairy whipped topping
2 teaspoons vanilla extract
3 tablespoons chocolate syrup

Beat egg whites (which are at room temperature) until stiff. Add sugar and continue to beat. Fold whipped topping into beaten egg whites; add vanilla and chocolate syrup. Spoon into 1-pint container. Freeze until firm.

NUTRIENTS, per serving:

Calories 252	Protein 4.5 gm	Carbohydrates 38 gm
Calcium 8 mg	Total fat 10 gm	Saturated fat 8 gm

EXCHANGES, not applicable

VANILLA ICE CREAM   *8 servings*

8 ounces non-dairy whipped topping
½ cup sugar
1 teaspoon vanilla extract
1 egg, separated

To the non-dairy topping add sugar, vanilla and egg yolk; blend then freeze for 30 minutes. In a small bowl, beat egg white (which is at room temperature) until stiff. Remove frozen mixture from freezer, fold in egg white and beat for 1 minute. Pour into plastic container, cover and freeze until firm .

NUTRIENTS, per serving:

Calories 190	Protein 0.2 gm	Carbohydrates 13 gm
Calcium 22 mg	Total fat 15 gm	Saturated fat 9 gm

EXCHANGES not applicable

STRAWBERRY ICE CREAM   *6 servings*

Cheese obtained from filtering 32 ounces of non-pasteurized yogurt
2 pints strawberries, washed, cleaned and crushed

In a bowl, place the yogurt cheese; add the strawberries; blend lightly and chill for several hours. Pour the mixture into a pan and freeze until firm; break into pieces and beat until smooth. Transfer into a chilled mold and freeze until firm.

NUTRIENTS, per serving:

Calories 111	Protein 8 gm	Carbohydrates 14 gm
Calcium 273 mg	Total fat 2.5 gm	Saturated fat 1.6 gm

EXCHANGES, per serving: 1 milk; ½ fat

MANDARIN ORANGE BAVARIAN   *4 servings*

1 package of orange gelatin (3 ounces)
1 can of mandarin oranges (11 ounces), with liquid
2 cups non-dairy whipped topping

Prepare the gelatin as directed on the package, using the liquid from the mandarin oranges in place of some of the required water. Cool. When the gelatin mixture is syrupy and partially set, fold in the mandarin oranges, then the whipped topping. Serve cold in parfait dishes.

NUTRIENTS, per serving:

Calories 183	Protein 2.4 gm	Carbohydrates 34 gm
Calcium 9 mg	Total fat 8 gm	Saturated fat 0.0 gm

EXCHANGES, not applicable

ORANGE BREAD PUDDING   *6 servings*

4 cups soy milk
3 tablespoons non-dairy margarine
2 cups dry, non-dairy bread cubes
½ cup sugar
2 eggs
1 teaspoon cinnamon
1 teaspoon nutmeg
1 orange rind, grated

Heat the milk and the margarine; when the margarine is melted, pour the mixture over the bread cubes. Let stand for a few minutes, then add the remaining ingredients. Pour this mixture into a greased 8-inch square baking dish, set in a pan of hot water and bake for 1 hour in a preheated 375° oven, or until a knife inserted in the center comes out clean. Serve hot or cold.

NUTRIENTS, per serving:

Calories 286	Protein 10 gm	Carbohydrates 36 gm
Calcium 75 mg	Total fat 11 gm	Saturated fat 1.5 gm

EXCHANGES, not applicable

RICE PUDDING

6 servings

1 cup white rice
4 cups water
2 tablespoons non-dairy margarine
4 tablespoons sugar
½ teaspoon vanilla extract
2 eggs
1/8 teaspoon cinnamon
2 tablespoons non-dairy cream

Cook rice according to package instructions. Add the margarine, sugar and vanilla, then fold in the beaten eggs. Bake in greased custard cups at 375° for 15 minutes; top with cinnamon and non-dairy cream.

NUTRIENTS, per serving:

Calories 160	Protein 2.7 gm	Carbohydrates 16.5 gm
Calcium 14 mg	Total fat 6.8 gm	Saturated fat 2.0 gm

EXCHANGES, not applicable

TAPIOCA PUDDING

2 servings

1½ tablespoons quick-cooking tapioca
1¼ cups lactose-reduced milk
¼ cup egg substitute
3 tablespoons sugar
½ teaspoon vanilla extract

Place the tapioca in a saucepan; add the milk slowly and stir; add the egg substitute and the sugar and cook at low heat for 10-12 minutes with stirring, until the mixture comes to a boil; add the vanilla. Pour into custard cups; serve hot or cold.

NUTRIENTS, per serving:

Calories 210	Protein 6 gm	Carbohydrates 36 gm
Calcium 150 mg	Total fat 5 gm	Saturated fat 4 gm

EXCHANGES, not applicable

CUSTARD PUDDING   *4 servings*

2 cups soy milk
1 tablespoon honey
1 teaspoon vanilla extract
1½ tablespoons cornstarch

Blend the first three ingredients in a saucepan; stir in the cornstarch, over a low flame, and continue stirring for 3 or 4 minutes until the pudding just begins to boil. Pour into custard cups. Garnish with drained fruit or crushed nuts. Serve chilled.

NUTRIENTS, per serving:

Calories 66	Protein 4 gm	Carbohydrates 10 gm
Calcium 150 mg	Total fat 5 gm	Saturated fat 4 gm

EXCHANGES, not applicable

BEVERAGES

Use of soy milks, tofu and/or non-dairy cream substitutes permit non-dairy drinks to be made that are "creamy" and nutritious.

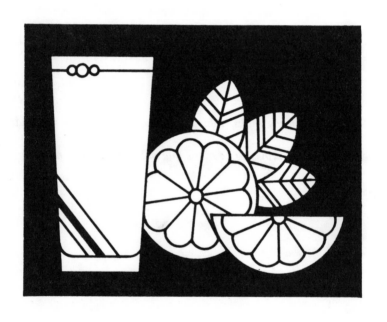

HAWAIIAN SHAKE

3 servings

1 cup soy milk
1 cup pineapple juice
4 ice cubes

Blend at high speed in a blender for a few seconds. The pineapple juice may be replaced by 1 cup orange juice or 2/3 cup cranberry juice.

NUTRIENTS, per serving:

Calories 64	Protein 3 gm	Carbohydrates 15 gm
Calcium 29 mg	Total fat 1.4 gm	Saturated fat 0.0 gm

EXCHANGES, per serving: ½ bread; ½ fruit

COFFEE FRAPPE

3 servings

1 cup soy milk
1 cup coffee, double strength
½ teaspoon sugar
4 ice cubes

Blend ingredients at high speed in a blender for a few seconds.

NUTRIENTS, per serving:

Calories 33	Protein 2.6 gm	Carbohydrates 4 gm
Calcium 18 mg	Total fat 1.2 gm	Saturated fat 0.0 gm

EXCHANGES, not applicable

FRUIT SHAKE   *3 servings*

1 cup soy milk
1 banana
2 ice cubes

Blend ingredients at high speed in a blender for a few seconds. In place of the banana, 1 cup canned apricots, 2 cups frozen raspberries, or 2½ cups frozen strawberries may be used.

NUTRIENTS, per serving:

Calories 64	Protein 3 gm	Carbohydrates 11 gm
Calcium 20.5 mg	Total fat 1.5 gm	Saturated fat 0.0 gm

EXCHANGES, per serving: 1 vegetable; ½ fruit

CREAMY FRUIT SHAKE   *4 servings*

10 ounces tofu, drained
1½ cups frozen strawberries
1 cup orange juice
4 ice cubes

Blend all ingredients at high speed in a blender for 5-10 seconds.

NUTRIENTS, per serving:

Calories 83	Protein 5 gm	Carbohydrates 11 gm
Calcium 86 mg	Total fat 2.6 gm	Saturated fat 0.5 gm

EXCHANGES, per serving: ½ fat; 1 vegetable; ½ fruit

CHOCOLATE SHAKE   *1 serving*

6 ounces soy milk
¼ teaspoon vanilla extract
2 heaping teaspoons non-dairy instant chocolate drink mix
4 ice cubes

Blend at high speed in a blender for a few seconds.

NUTRIENTS, per serving:

Calories 208	Protein 7 gm	Carbohydrates 24 gm
Calcium 47 mg	Total fat 1 gm	Saturated fat 4 gm

EXCHANGES, not applicable

CHOCOLATE "EGG CREAM"   *1 serving*

¼ cup soy milk
3 tablespoons non-dairy chocolate syrup
8 ounces seltzer water (or club soda)

Add the syrup to a tall glass; add the soy milk (do not stir yet). Pour in the carbonated water and stir.

NUTRIENTS, per serving:

Calories 220	Protein 2.6 gm	Carbohydrates 40 gm
Calcium 24 mg	Total fat 6.5 gm	Saturated fat 0.0 gm

EXCHANGES, not applicable

SELECTED

BIBLIOGRAPHY

The references given offer the interested reader additional information about lactose-sensitivity -- discussions ranging from the philosophy of the ailment to the listings of manufacturers of lactose-free products.

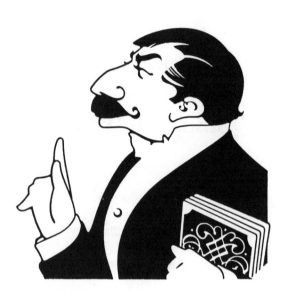

Diagnosis and Treatment of Lactose Intolerance. <u>Brit. Med. J.</u> 286/6304 pgs 1423-1424 (1981)

Effectiveness of Milk Products in Management of Lactose Malabsorption. <u>Am. J. Clin. Nutr.</u> 34/12 pgs 2711-2715 (1981)

Treatment of Lactose Intolerance. <u>Med. Lett. Drug. Ther.</u> 23/15 pgs 67-68 (1981)

Cause, Diagnosis and Chemotherapy of Lactose Intolerance. <u>Br. Med. J.</u> 284/6326 pgs 1405 (1982)

Lactose Malabsorption and Tolerance of Lactose-Hydrolyzed Milk. <u>Scand. J. Gastrointerol.</u> 17/7 pgs 861-864 (1982)

The Allergic Gourmet. <u>Contemporary Books, Inc.</u> 294 pgs (1983)

Congenital Lactose Deficiency. <u>Arch. Dis. Child.</u> 58/4 pgs 246-252 (1983)

Primary Lactose Intolerance in Zulu Adults. <u>S. Afr. Med. G.</u> 63/20 pgs 778-780 (1983)

Enzyme Replacement Therapy for Primary Adult Lactose Deficiency. <u>Gastroenterology</u> 87/5 pgs 1072-1082 (1984)

Lactose Malabsorption from Yogurts and Treated Milks. <u>Am. G. Clin. Nutr.</u> 40/6 pgs 1219-1223 (1984)

Food Sensitivity. <u>The American Dietetic Association.</u> 127 pgs (1985)

Lactose Intolerance. <u>The American Dietetic Association.</u> 77 pgs (1985)

Nutritional Implications of Lactose and Lactose Activity. <u>Dairy Council Digest.</u> 56/5 pgs 25-30 (1985)

For Want of Lactose. <u>Am. J. Nurs.</u> 86/8 pgs 902-906 (1986)

Lactose Deficiency and Lactose Malabsorption. <u>Z. Gastrointerol.</u> 24/3 pgs 125-134 (1986)

Lactose Malabsorption and Intolerance in Italians. <u>Dig. Dis. Sci.</u> 31/12 pgs 1313-1316 (1986)

Handbook of Food Allergies. <u>Midwest Immunology Center, Galesburg, MI.</u> 320 pgs (1986)

The Milk Sugar Dilemma: Living with Lactose Intolerance. <u>Medi-Ed Press, East Lansing, MI.</u> 256 pgs (1987)

Lactose Intolerance: Translating Research Information. <u>Summary of NDC Nutrition Research Conference.</u> 9 pgs (1987)

Dairy-Free Cookbook. <u>Prima Publishing and Communications, Rocklin, CA.</u> 322 pgs (1989)

INDEX

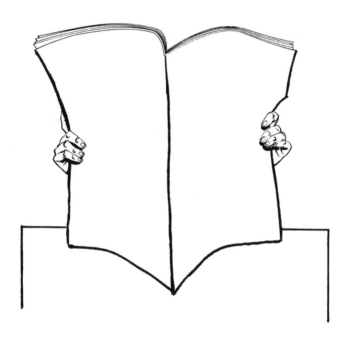

ORDER FORM

Please send me _____ copy(ies) of Lactose-Free Cooking at $14.00 each, tax and postage included.

I understand that I may return the book within 10 days for a full refund if I'm not satisfied.

Name: _____

Address: _____

State & Zip: _____

Amount Enclosed: _____

Check _____   *Money Order* _____

Mail Order to: Lockley Publishing Company
P O Box 3263
Wayne, New Jersey 07474 3263